Beyond Stuttering

The McGuire Programme for Getting Good at the
Sport of Speaking

Dave McGuire

Souvenir Press

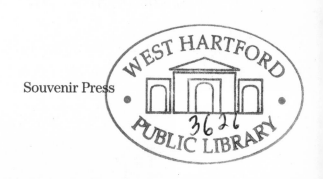

The McGuire Programme California LLC
Email: dave@mcguireprogramme.com
Web Site: www.mcguireprogramme.com
Copyright no. TXu 804 545
United States Library of Congress

First published under the title *Beyond Stammering*
in Great Britain in 2003 by Souvenir Press Ltd
43 Great Russell Street, London WC1B 3PD

A revised edition of *Beyond Stammering* was published 2008.
Reprinted 4 times.

This revised and updated edition under the title
Beyond Stuttering published 2014
Reprinted 2015 (twice), 2016

ISBN 978 02856 42843

Typeset by M Rules

Printed and bound by CPI Group (UK) Ltd, Croydon, CR0 4YY

This book is dedicated to my children, my parents and all those who participated in our mission to help people who stutter throughout the world. I would like to give special thanks to Maria McGrath, Chris Cooksey, Joe O'Donnell, Niels van de Kreeke and Sean Rees for their help with editing, formatting and graphics, and to those many others who have contributed to this book. Special thanks, too, to Dr. Ron Kapp who organized our first intensive course.

Preface

About myself and the Programme

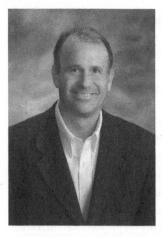

In 1969, after trying several forms of therapy, I had a chance to defeat my severe stutter with the help of Dr. Joe Sheehan. At the time he was a psychology professor at UCLA and considered to be one of the very best stuttering therapists in the world. His Programme was based on active non-avoidance and acceptance of oneself as a stutterer. Although my speech had improved and I was able to develop a career in adolescent psychology, my lack of discipline and downright laziness resulted in many severe relapses that devastated my personal and professional life. In critical moments when I really needed to speak well, the words would not come.

In November 1993, after 24 more wasted years, I was given another chance in a Diaphragm training Programme developed by a famous opera singer in Amsterdam. Although this Diaphragm training resulted in a strong, immediate fluency where I thought for sure I was 'cured', I relapsed after a couple of weeks. Having attained the impossible then losing it was devastating and, like a runaway slave being caught by his master, the fear returned with a vengeance. Thankfully, I was able to use Joe Sheehan's concepts to bring the fear down to where I could use (what I now know to be) Costal Diaphragmatic Breathing to get back my strong, rather articulate and eloquent way of speaking. From this I realized that this would not be the magic pill we who stutter dream about, but an ongoing lifelong process very much like any skilled sport or performing art.

Not cured because I still have to work at it, but being able to speak well and being proud of the way I speak in very challenging situations is very much worth the time and effort. Shortly after I 'got it', and having had already created a very successful Adolescent treatment Programme in the USA, I figured I could start a Programme for those who stutter using a combination of Costal Diaphragm training, non-avoidance/role-conflict resolution, and various methods from Sports Psychology.

In February 1994, the McGuire Programme became a reality as a few brave stutterers took a chance and worked with me at my house in Holland. Soon, the successful ones (the ones who worked hard, were courageous and persevered) were spreading the word in their own countries, arranging courses for me to instruct, and inviting the 'veterans' to come help coach the new ones.

By 1995 the Programme evolved from 'my' to 'our' as more members became Coaches, Course Instructors, Staff Trainers and Regional Directors organizing courses and providing critical follow-up support throughout the world. Our regions are currently established in the United Kingdom, Ireland, USA, Australia, New Zealand, Holland/Belgium, Scandinavia, South Africa, Mexico, Spain/Portugal, India, and the Middle East (Dubai).

Dave McGuire

Contents

Foreword

By John Harrison

My first encounter with Dave McGuire and the McGuire Programme took place at the Fourth International Conference for People who Stutter, held in Linköping, Sweden, during the summer of 1995. As we chatted about common interests, I learned that Dave had previously run an innovative Programme for teenage boys with behavioral problems. Back in the 60s I had been an active sponsor of a similar kind of residential Programme for drug addicts. Both of us had seen that the only way to effect lasting behavioral change was to address the entire person.

Dave's approach to stuttering combines his training in psychology with other stuttering therapies and sports psychology. Into the mix also went the know-how gained from his experience of working with difficult teenagers. This eclectic background accounts, in part, for the uniqueness of the McGuire Programme. It's also sets Dave apart from most others working in the field of stuttering remediation.

At the end of our initial conversation, Dave asked whether I would like to stop by and observe a demonstration of his Programme run with several of his graduates. I would indeed, and off we went to his workshop. My first impression of the workshop is still etched in memory – a group of men and women in a circle taking deep breaths with belts strapped around their chests. What in the world were they doing? I wasn't sure what to make of it, but I was really curious. During further conversations at the conference, it became clear that Dave and I shared a common view of stuttering, and we promised to stay in touch once the conference was over.

I was intrigued with the McGuire Programme. As someone who had stuttered for roughly 30 years and who had made a full and lasting recovery, I saw a recovery strategy similar to what I, myself, had followed. As an émigré to California from New York in the early 1960s, I had immersed myself in the personal growth movement that was flourishing on America's west coast. I'd grown up with a very fuzzy image of myself and needed to change many beliefs and behaviors that did not serve me well. In working to build self-esteem and get my own house in order, something very interesting happened: my stuttering gradually slipped away.

According to most speech therapists, this was not supposed to happen. The prevailing belief was 'once a stutterer, always a stutterer'. But that was evidently not true, at least for some people. Over time, I saw that my stuttering was not simply a product of bad speech behaviors, it was also a reflection of who I was as an individual – how I thought and felt, how I functioned, what I believed. My speech blocks had everything to do with the system of self that I had created, a system that supported a dysfluent way of speaking. Therefore, to make permanent changes in my speech, I had to address a total system that included my emotions, perceptions, beliefs, intentions, and speech behaviors. And it all had to be brought into alignment.

What so intrigued me about the McGuire Programme was that this was the first Programme I'd encountered that took a broad, holistic approach to stuttering and that touched on many of the same issues that I had addressed in my own recovery. Not only did the McGuire Method focus on the speech process itself, it also focused on the underlying factors that supported the stuttering behavior. Even today, several characteristics of the Programme are truly unusual.

- The Programme uses Costal breathing to keep the breath open and prevent speech blocks. The Programme focuses not just on 'can I speak' but on 'how do I want to speak?' Eloquence is a stop on the path to fluency.
- Members do the teaching and coaching – there is no professional staff of speech therapists – giving teeth to the concepts

that (1) the real experts are those who have personally worked through the problem, and (2) best way to learn something is to teach it to others.

- McGuire also has the best long-term follow-up Programme in the world. It is free and open ended. Coaches and those being coached routinely connect by phone and email and those connections often reach half way around the world.
- A member can attend any number of intensive courses, support groups, and/or refresher days for just a very small token fee.
- Members are free to suggest changes to the course, which accounts for the fact that the McGuire Programme continues to evolve.

This book will be useful to anyone who wants to gain a clear and detailed picture of what is involved in the recovery process. As you'll discover, the road will take you through more than just changes in how to speak and how to manage speech blocks. It will help bring to awareness the subtle ways in which you've shaped your world to support your stuttering. You'll also acquire a better sense of those issues that need to be addressed in order to break through into a newer, freer way of speaking.

You'll learn, not just about how to acquire fluency, but how to *keep* it. You'll develop an understanding of the various factors that trigger relapses – why they happen, and what to do about them.

The text is full of sports analogies – highly appropriate, considering that speaking, like tennis, is a performance skill and subject to many of the same pressures and pitfalls. You'll be introduced to various practice techniques needed to etch new speech behaviors into your psyche, and you'll be offered various recovery strategies that you can fall back on when you run into turbulence and slip into relapse.

Finally, you'll gain a perspective on the 'life games' that can either undermine or support your progress.

Can you overcome stuttering just by reading this book? That's like asking, 'Can you get from London to Bath by simply reading a roadmap?' In both cases, the answer is 'not likely'. If you want to get from point A to point B, you need to put yourself in motion, commit yourself to the journey, and decide you won't quit until you reach your destination. Some people have the discipline to make the trip themselves. Others will want assistance, either from a speech therapist, or by enrolling in one of the trainings presented by the McGuire Programme in various countries. But whatever your choice, this book is an excellent 'map' that will help you proceed on your journey better informed and with a clearer set of objectives.

Since 1995, I have been privileged to meet many members of the McGuire Programme, and I have observed several 4-day trainings in their entirety. I've heard the members' stories. I've seen the results. What is clear is that overcoming a stutter is, for most, a difficult and challenging trip. It requires persistence, a clear commitment, a strong sense of dedication, and a willingness to repeatedly step outside your comfort zone.

But given a hearty resolve, it is also clear that the Programme works. I invite you to open your mind and allow yourself to discover a total approach to the age-old problem of chronic stuttering.

Bio: **John C. Harrison** is no stranger to the problems of stuttering. He showed a marked dysfluency at the age of three and two years later underwent therapy at the National Hospital for Speech and Hearing Disorders in New York City. But this and later efforts at therapy during his school years were not successful and he struggled with stuttering throughout college and well into adulthood.

Harrison's involvement in a broad variety of personal growth Programmes over three decades have given him a unique insight into the nature and dynamics of the stuttering person. Today, he is fully recovered and no longer deals with a stuttering problem.

One of the earliest members of the National Stuttering Association, Harrison was an 18-year member of the Board of Directors and is currently the editor of the NSA's monthly newsletter *Letting Go*. Harrison has run workshops for the stuttering and the professional communities across the U.S. and Canada as well as in Ireland, the U.K., and Australia. He has been published in *Advance Magazine* and the *Journal of Fluency Disorders* and has presented at conventions of the American Speech Language Hearing Association and the California Speech Language Hearing Association, as well as at the First World Congress on Fluency Disorders in Munich, Germany.

Harrison lives with his wife, Doris, a graphic designer, in San Francisco where he works as a freelance writer.

Introduction

This book started out in 1994 as the manual for a world-wide Programme known as 'The McGuire Programme,™ Freedom's Road®'. It is an association of regional Programmes owned and instructed by people who are in the process of going from people who stutter uncontrollably, to people who enjoy speaking and do it well. Our mission is to help other people who stutter throughout the world.

In 2001 I was approached by Souvenir Press to make this available to the public. So here it is ... but with some cautions:

This book is *not* for those who are satisfied with the constraints dictated by stuttering. Nor is it for those looking for a permanent cure. We cannot guarantee that you will never stutter again any more than any tennis camp could guarantee even the world's number one tennis player that he will never again double fault or blow an easy shot. It is a way, if you're willing to work hard and be courageous, to become an articulate, even eloquent speaker, and have fun playing this wonderful sport of verbal communication.

You should also know that this will indeed be very much like learning a skilled sport such as tennis or skiing from a book. If you're talented and persistent with a good work ethic, and courage, you can probably make significant progress. Chances are, however, you would need help from a qualified tennis/ski instructor. Same with the sport of speaking. Although some people can make significant improvements in their speech through this book, most will need personal instruction.

If you try this on your own, give it six months of your best effort. If there is significant progress, then keep going. If your gut tells you this is the right path, you've sincerely done your best, but you are not happy with the progress, it probably means that you need coaching and follow-up support. Contact us, then, through our website: www.mcguireprogramme.com and apply to join our Programme.

PART ONE:

How to get it

*Most of the important things in the world
have been accomplished by people who have
kept on trying when there seemed
to be no hope at all.*
DALE CARNEGIE

'Getting it' is like any other significant accomplishment. You
are better off having goals and objectives.

OUR GOAL: Articulate Eloquence ... *'Playing to win'*

Ultimately, your goal is to become an eloquent as well as articulate
speaker rather than simply a 'non-stutterer'. As in sports psychology this requires developing the mentality of 'playing to win' rather
than 'playing not to lose'. To be articulate is to pronounce each
sound how it is meant to be pronounced. It also includes things like
conciseness, inflection and clarity. Add to this passion and truth-
fulness for what you're saying and you've reached 'eloquence'. To
achieve this, we have the following objectives:

Physically: to counteract the freezing, struggle and distortion that
happens in the Diaphragm, Vocal Cords, and Articulators during the
stuttering block and learn to speak powerfully from the Thorax
using the Costal Diaphragm and other techniques.

Mentally: there are six objectives:

- To understand the dynamics of stuttering.
- To counteract the tendency to 'hold back' and use avoidance mechanisms.
- To deal with the fear.
- To accept yourself as someone working hard to overcome stuttering and having to go through various stages of improvement.
- To develop an assertive attitude to attack your feared words and situations.
- To understand the process of losing what you've gained and how to counteract it.

Emotionally: once you have dealt with the fear, the objective is to let go and *have fun* speaking.

Spiritually: the objective is self-actualization. Once your verbal self is set free, who will be doing the talking? Are you the person you want to be? These positive internal changes – beliefs, intentions, perceptions, etc. – are necessary to attain and hold on to articulate eloquence.

CHAPTER ONE:

Understanding the mental and emotional part of stuttering

Before we can start to do something about your stutter, we need to have a basic understanding of at least one theory of what it's all about. This chapter is about the mental and emotional part. The next chapter will get into the physical part. Then, in the third chapter, you'll get what you need to become a good speaker.

Volumes have been written about stuttering, the cause of which has not been proven. Some say it's genetic. Others say it's the result of a neurological defect. Others say it's purely psychological. Nothing has been proven scientifically. For purposes of doing something about it, although admittedly unscientific, our belief is that it follows the dynamics of behavior and sports psychology, and results in physical dysfunctions that in turn intensify the psychological and ends up in a vicious cycle.

By 'psychology', we mean the mental, emotional and attitudinal factors involved. For the most part it is the same thing that musicians and athletes go through when they are afraid to make a mistake. It's called:

'Choking'

You can see it as 'performance fear' gone wild. You see it during penalty kicks at important soccer matches. It's relatively easy for a good kicker to make a goal from that distance even against the best of goalies. But how many times have you soccer fans seen the ball sail high or wide? And you KNOW that what is going on in the kicker's head is 'better not blow it!'

Or the tennis player who blows the easy shot or double faults away a point that would win the match or get him or her back in the game. Or the trumpet player who misses the high note during a performance. Or the field goal kicker in American Football blowing a point he can make with his eyes closed in practice. Or the pro golfer missing the easy putt.

For us who stutter, it is the fear of stuttering – of blowing getting out that word. More accurately, the fear of being seen as someone who stutters.

The multi approach-avoidance conflict: 'Kangaroo in the headlights.'

One Australian member of our Programme came up with this one to explain how he felt during a stuttering block. Kangaroo starts across the road, sees the car/headlights coming, can't decide whether to keep going across the road, or go back. So he freezes in the road.

It best describes a dynamic, which comes from some very basic experiments in behaviorist psychology, mostly BF Skinner, where rats were put in cages with food at one end. But there was a catch. There was also an electric grid, so that every time the rats tried to get the food, they were given electric shocks. The rats wanted the food, but were afraid of the shock. This came to be known as the 'single approach avoidance conflict'.

Now, take those same rats and put another food and shock at the other end of the box. Here you have a double approach-avoidance conflict. Put other lanes in the cage with the same reward and punishment at each end, and you have a 'multiple approach-avoidance conflict'. The more lanes, the more stressed the rats become. Sort of like that kangaroo getting caught in the headlights in a busy intersection.

Same with people. The more unresolved choices, the higher the stress. It could be argued that the more unresolved conflicts we have, the more dysfunctional we are. Perhaps mental health simply boils down to how quickly and effectively we can resolve our Approach-Avoidance conflicts.

How does this apply to stuttering? In a single approach avoidance conflict, the desire for food is *the desire to be perceived as fluent.* The fear of an electric shock is the *fear of being perceived as a stutterer.* But, with those who stutter, it is seldom a single approach-avoidance conflict. Those conflicts, which we share with fluent speakers, become turbo-charged by our stuttering. Here are a few of the biggies:

The fear of being too slow versus desire to communicate quickly: One problem with stuttering is that it takes more time to speak. Especially with children, many people don't want to wait and will be obvious with their impatience.

Fear of disrespect versus desire for respect: This applies to when you are dealing with someone whose perceived social status is higher than yours. But not always, it can apply to teenagers and children – anyone from whom you want respect. It is difficult to get this respect with an out-of-control stutter.

Fear of being perceived as incompetent versus desire to be perceived as competent: In business or formal social situations, you want the other people to see you as competent in whatever you are doing. When dealing with a nasty block while trying to explain something to customers, colleagues, etc. some folks will perceive you as incompetent.

Fear of not speaking versus desire to shut up: Sometimes you don't want to speak with anyone. You want to be left alone. Then some bored turkey bursts into your office wanting to chat. Or your sister-in-law comes over right before your Sunday afternoon nap. You don't want to communicate, but you're afraid not to.

Fear of being perceived as insane versus desire to be perceived as sane: A stutterer using lots of tricks and avoidances no longer looks like a stutterer. People understand stuttering. They don't understand jaw chomping, leg slapping, tongue thrusts, and head jerking. Some folks will see it as crazy.

Fear of rejection versus desire for acceptance: Almost everyone wants social acceptance. Almost nobody wants to be rejected. Especially with potential love relationships. The more approach-avoidance conflicts, the more severe the stutter.

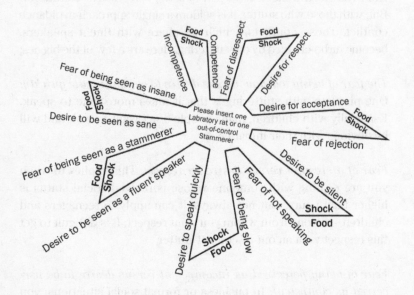

Not your usual fear-based choking

The pattern is the same, but there are some notable differences between performance fear-based choking of sports and music, and that of stuttering. Although one can cite many examples of young athletes and musicians being bullied by parents and coaches for failure, the humiliation and trauma experienced by a person who stutters (especially youngsters) is infinitely more intense and the psychological damage more severe. An athlete or musician does not need to do the sport or music to feel part of the human race. But the person who stutters can't do a very basic, necessary function that very young kids can do so easily. There is a huge difference between Johnny who can't make a free throw in basketball, and Teddy who stands there in front of the class trying for 5 minutes to get through a simple sentence.

Then, there is the dynamic that sometimes, on a cursed 'good day', even the worst person who stutters can be quite fluent. Problem is the people around him are thinking, 'There! See! He CAN do it. Just has to put his mind to it and stop being lazy.' Then the next day comes, things are going bad, words won't come regardless of the struggle and number of tricks being used, and those around the young person who stutters give the message covertly or overtly of 'What's the matter with you!? You were talking perfectly yesterday.' Pressure to perform increases.

Young athletes who have been abused have the option of 'getting out of Dodge' at some point. In other words, they can stop playing their sport or musical instrument when they are at an age to stand up to adults and make their own decisions. Not so with stuttering people. We can't dump our rackets or trombone into the garbage and walk away. We *have* to speak (and speak reasonably well) to prosper in society. We *have* to play this sport.

The cycle of panic

It can be argued that most psychological things tend to run in cycles. With stuttering it can best be described as a Cycle of Panic. Not just fear. Not just anxiety. Panic.

Starting with:

Performance fear: This is tied into fear of failure, which specifically is tied to the fear of stuttering, or, more precisely, the fear of being seen as a person who stutters. It leads to:

Confusion: You don't know where to go, what to do. It's like walking through a minefield not knowing if you'll get blown up with your next step. By adding this confusion to the fear, you start getting into the realm of panic, which leads to:

Holding back: Someone going through a minefield not knowing where the mines are will hold back on taking that next step, or inch their way through. When this fear of stepping on a mine becomes great enough, everything freezes up and the person is caught in the:

Approach-avoidance conflict: Or the mental block. Can't go forward, can't go backwards. Stuck. If, for the person who stutters, there is no escape or resolution, he experiences what is commonly known as a:

Physical 'Block': All those muscles starting with the Diaphragm, then those muscles controlling the vocal cords and articulators freeze then, many times, struggle and distort. Then here come the various tricks and attempts to avoid. The delivery of the word, just like the flubbed extra point kick, is blown and the person who stutters experiences:

Shame, Self-hate, Guilt: But a very intense version. Because we cannot stop speaking, we people who stutter develop various mechanisms and struggles to avoid the act of stuttering by substituting words, slapping legs, biting tongues, cutting off sounds, etc. Although these might get the feared word out part way through the minefield of the speaking situation, the act of avoiding (running away), which many times makes the struggling stutter seem bizarre, increases the original performance fear.

Unless a miracle happens, or some kind of strong intervention, this cycle repeats itself, becoming more intense each time (increasing the severity of that mish-mash of freezing, struggle, distortion, tricks and avoidance called 'stuttering') until the situation ends.

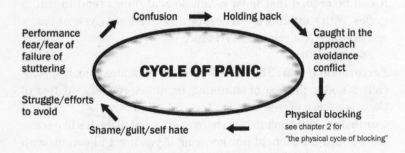

But that's not the end of it. The memory of this sticks around for the next difficult speaking situation where it raises its not-so-pretty head, taps you on the shoulder and whispers in your ear 'remember what happened the last time …?'

Roots of the fear

My personal recollection of myself as a severely stuttering young junior high school student standing before a class of Victorville street thugs, enduring their merciless teasing while trying to deliver the dreaded 'oral report' – and the hours or days leading up to it – was that death would have been much preferable. I often wondered why the fear of stuttering is so overwhelming. Why is it so important to speak clearly? What's so bad about stuttering?

Being different: Breaking it down, the simple answer is that it makes us different. But in a negative way. We're different because we are, many times, seen as incompetent. After all, speaking (reasonably well) is so easy. Little kids can do it without even thinking, like walking down the street. We are seen as incompetent because sometimes we can speak fluently. It's just when the pressure is on that we fall apart. It's like someone who needs crutches to walk suddenly being able to run and dance and play tennis, then, just because something upsets him, can't take two steps without the crutches. Now we've added a major mental weakness or even insanity to what was perceived as a 'physical' problem.

Need for Perfection: Let's face it. The more perfect we are in this society, the more goodies we get. So the desire to be good-looking, look young, have a great body, be intelligent and educated, be rich, have a big house and impressive cars etc. is overwhelming. You hear from pop psychologists that we need to love and accept others and ourselves regardless of the faults, but the reality is still that we are judged by what we DO and how well we do it. We shouldn't 'be' what we do, but the reality is that we indeed 'are' what we do. Factor into this not being able to do that very basic thing called 'talking' and the fear of not being perfect versus the desire to be perfect is very strong.

Alone: It would appear that for at least thousands of years, we survived as herd creatures. A predator, if it meant to do harm to one member, would have to deal with the whole mob. To be 'different' meant risking rejection from the tribe or clan. Such rejection meant the possibility of being cast out into the wilderness alone without the protection of the herd.

Then you have the very basic need to find a mate and procreate. Unless being different led to being an innovative leader or, say, inventing something new and useful to the clan, those who did not measure up to the normal standards found it very hard to find a mate. Probably more true for males than for females when it came/comes to stuttering, which is probably why there are so many more males who stutter than females.

Figure we evolved for generations with this fear of rejection and being alone and not 'qualifying' for a mate. Apply it to a young person struggling ALONE through an oral report in class and you get the picture. This 'sense of isolation', that you're the only one on the planet with this problem, can be overwhelming and turn fear into panic.

One of the most effective things about the McGuire Programme is the support system. We learned early on that even the best technique or method is ineffective without support from others with the same goal that addresses this fear of being alone (sense of isolation).

Persecution: Add to this such practices as branding or cutting out pieces of the tongues of people who stutter in the Middle Ages that might very well go back for millennia. If Karl Jung's theories of the 'collective human consciousness' or even the theories of reincarnation that such trauma gets passed on from generation to generation is valid, you have another deep-seated source of fear and panic.

Covert and overt stuttering

There are two types of people who stutter: one type is very successful at hiding the stutter by skillful use of tricks and word substitution and situation avoidance. We refer to these folks as 'coverts'. Many times those who he or she has known for years do not know that they stutter. But a successful covert person who stutters is going through life living in a minefield waiting for the ax to fall ... waiting for that situation they can't get out of, or there just isn't another word to substitute for the word they know will cause a big embarrassing block.

In many ways, a covert person who stutters will have a tougher time because it is relatively easy to go back to tricks and avoidance that have kept up the façade of normal speaking. Someone who is an overt stutterer is simply an unsuccessful covert stutterer. They try to avoid and use tricks, but the struggle and blocking is there for everyone to see. Perhaps they were successful for a while at hiding the stutter, but ran into a few too many unavoidable, untrickable, inescapable words and situations, which caused them to lose confidence in their hiding/avoiding strategies and panic started to rule the day. Coverts are better than overts at controlling the panic.

Generally, the worse the stutter, or more overt, the better. Things can only get better. You tend to get much support from those around you when improvement is starting to be observable. You're not faced with the daunting task of the covert person who stutters of explaining to friends, associates, (and sometimes family) that you do indeed have a stuttering problem, which is the critical first foundational step.

For more insight into covert stuttering, read 'Battling' by the Irish graduate and instructor, Patrick Merrigan in the last section of this book.

You are what you resist

It is very true for those who stutter. All the struggle that you see on the surface of an overt person who stutters and under the surface of a covert person who stutters is fueled by efforts not to stutter. The more you resist being a person who stutters, the more you maintain the identity of a person who stutters.

'Then why try to become a fluent speaker' you ask? There is a big difference between trying not to stutter, and trying to speak well. In sports psychology, *it's the difference between playing to win and playing not to lose.* It is a matter of mental focus. Someone trying not to lose a tennis match, or not to stutter, is focusing on those things that cause poor performance. Someone 'playing to win' (or trying to be an effective, articulate, eloquent speaker) is focusing on those things that improve performance.

CHAPTER TWO:

The physical factor

Nothing in life is to be feared.
It is only to be understood.
MARIE CURIE 1867–1934

Whether you buy our belief in the psychology of stuttering or someone else's, its manifestation is some kind of physical behavior.
Something less than productive happens to those muscles that produce the spoken word as a result of the approach-avoidance
conflicts, cycle of panic, and avoidance mechanisms.

Enough research has been done to verify that the physical
dynamics of a stuttering block involves dysfunctions of breathing,
vocalizing, and/or articulating. Of these, we believe the most significant contributor to and possibly the physical precipitator of the
stuttering block – and the least attended to in most other therapies – is breathing. The main organ responsible for this dysfunction
is a muscle called the Diaphragm.

Some basic breathing anatomy

Let's start with the torso, which is all that area above the hips and
below the neck. Your torso is divided into two chambers: The
Abdomen, that area below the Diaphragm, and above the hip; and
the Thorax, which is the area above the Diaphragm below the neck
also known as the chest.

Actually, there are three chambers because the Thorax is divided
into two separate breathing chambers. These two breathing cham-

bers that house the lungs are actually vacuum chambers. The main mechanism for operating these vacuum chambers is the Diaphragm, which also divides the Thorax from the abdomen.

When it's time to take a breath of air, the brain sends a message to the Diaphragm to contract. When the Diaphragm contracts, it becomes smaller and the top, called the 'central tendon,' moves towards the Abdomen. This creates more space in the chest cavities, which creates a vacuum. Just like pulling the plunger out on a bicycle pump. Air rushes in and fills the little air sacks (Alveoli) in the lungs.

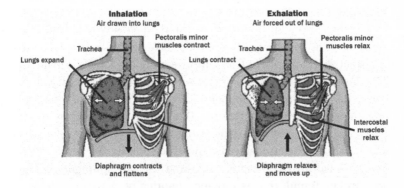

When it's time to breathe out or speak, the Diaphragm relaxes therefore becoming bigger and moving deeper into the Thorax. This means less space in the Thorax. Less space means less vacuum. Less vacuum means the air goes out of the lungs.

The Diaphragm

Now that you have the big picture of the breathing mechanism, let's talk about the Diaphragm itself. It is shaped like a huge bell in the Thorax. The heart sits right in the middle and is attached to the Diaphragm by the same membrane that lines the torso.

Under the left lobe of the Diaphragm is the stomach. Under the right lobe is the liver.

The Diaphragm is one of the biggest muscles in the body, and *the* biggest semi-automatic muscle in the body. Semi-automatic means that it operates much like your eyelashes – part of its function you have no conscious control over, part you do have conscious control over. This is mainly so that you can keep on breathing while you're asleep. It is also so that you can do other things than having constantly to think: 'Okay, now, on the count of three, breathe in, breathe out, breathe in, breathe out' all day long. That would be almost as bad as having consciously to think about flipping television channels.

All muscles are to a certain extent involuntary. Just watch what you do the next time someone yells at you unexpectedly. Your arms fly up to cover your face, or your chest, or your groin. What are your muscles doing? They are contracting. They are preparing to protect, or to fight, or to run away. And, of course, you also inhale sharply.

Now why do you suppose you would inhale sharply? Well, it is because your Diaphragm is a muscle. Like all muscles, it tends to contract as a response to fear. Unfortunately, the Diaphragm needs to relax in order to speak. You have two powerful forces trying to move the Diaphragm in opposite directions. You have the natural response to fear contracting the Diaphragm and drawing air in. Then you have your own desire to speak trying to relax the Diaphragm so that air can move over the vocal cords. The result is what? A frozen Diaphragm, of course. Or a Diaphragm, as one researcher found, that is moving chaotically. A frozen, chaotic Diaphragm means no airflow or chaotic airflow. No airflow means no speech. Chaotic airflow means ... well chaotic speech. Both can be symptom of that phenomenon called stuttering.

'Home of the Soul': The ancient Greeks called the Diaphragm 'the home of the soul' because the nerve that controls the Diaphragm is called the Phrenic nerve – Phrenic is the Greek word for soul. Homer even referred to it as the home of the emotions. I suspect he was right. Don't know about you, but when I'm angry I feel it in my chest. When I'm crying, there may be tears coming out of my eyes, but the feeling is in my chest. When I laugh, you may hear it from my mouth, but I feel it in my chest. When I'm afraid, I may have sweat running from my face, but I feel it in my chest.

Then the ancient Greeks had a word that sounds like 'Exphrenos', which means to speak from the emotions. We would probably translate that today as 'speaking from the heart.'

Assuming for now that the Diaphragm is the physical center of our emotions, it becomes more than an ordinary muscle reacting to fear by contracting. It is the muscle where we feel the emotion of fear. Add to this the fact we cannot see the Diaphragm functioning, and we begin to see why stuttering is such a mysterious affliction.

The two structures of the diaphragm: crural and costal

Before, I referred to the Diaphragm as one big muscle that controls breathing by controlling the vacuum in the two chambers of the Thorax. In terms of control of the crown (central tendon) of the Diaphragm, this is true; however, this crown is controlled by two separate sets of muscles. These two 'parts', 'Crural' and 'Costal', and can function so independently from each other that some experts on the Diaphragm refer to these, as we will throughout this book, as the 'Crural Diaphragm' and the 'Costal Diaphragm' although they are officially two parts of the same structure.

Crural part of the diaphragm ('crural diaphragm'): This structure of the Diaphragm is attached to the spine. When it contracts, it displaces your abdomen in order to make room for the vacuum in your Thorax to draw in air. This is functioning when your tummy is moving in and out when you breathe. If your chest happens to move up and down, it is a secondary result of the abdomen displacement.

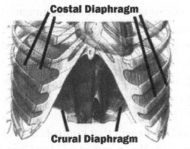

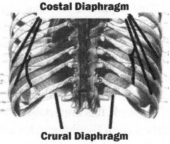

Front view of the Thorax   Rear view of the Thorax

The Crural Diaphragm is responsible for probably 98% of your breathing.

It is what operates when you are sleeping and when your body doesn't need a lot of air. It therefore operates mostly automatically. Most folks speak from air produced by the Crural Diaphragm.

Costal part of the diaphragm ('costal diaphragm'): Looking at the pictures, you can see that the Costal Diaphragm is much larger than the Crural part of the Diaphragm ('Crural Diaphragm'). It is attached to the bottom of the ribs. When the Costal Diaphragm contracts, the rib cage also pulls up and out expanding the volume of the Thorax to create a vacuum. (Whether the Costal Diaphragm plays a role in pulling the ribs up and out is unknown, but, for sure, you know that the Costal Diaphragm is being used when the ribs are expanding.)

You know your Costal Diaphragm is working when you yawn. Body is just asking for more oxygen. It is also used during heavy exercise, heavy coughing and sneezing. You also use it sometimes when you shout or sing loudly. Its action is usually voluntary – you have control over when it is used or not used.

In 1962, the world's leading expert on the Diaphragm, Dr. Peter Macklem of McGill University in Canada, did a study to determine the various functions of the Diaphragm. A dog (respiratory function basically the same as in humans) was hooked up to electrodes where the C5 C6 and C7 nerve roots (corresponding to C3, C4, C5, in humans) could be individually stimulated. All these roots join into the phrenic nerve, which then branches into two parts above the heart. The right branch goes to the Crural Diaphragm and the left into the Costal Diaphragm.

What happened was that when the dog's C7 root was stimulated, *only* the Crural Diaphragm contracted. When the C5 was stimulated, *only* the Costal Diaphragm contracted and the ribs expanded, which meant there was also some interaction with the Inter-costal muscles. When the C6 nerve root was stimulated, both parts of the Diaphragms contracted and ribs expanded.

So why is this important to you? Well, go back to the description of the Crural Diaphragm. It is this Diaphragm that controls the air-flow for normal speaking. From this we theorize that it is the Crural Diaphragm that is chronically contracting in response to fear in those who stutter.

Now, we can retrain the Crural Diaphragm for years to counteract this chronic contracting during speech. Or we can spend years desensitizing ourselves to the fear. Or we can do it quicker by bypassing the Crural Diaphragm and going to the Costal Diaphragm and its separate nerves.

Many stutterers who have trained themselves to speak from the Costal Diaphragm have overcome stuttering and now consider themselves to be articulate, even eloquent, speakers. Why? Perhaps for two reasons. First, is that you become a more powerful speaker for the same reason an opera singer sings better using the Costal Diaphragm. Secondly, if the Diaphragm is the home of the emotions, by focusing on this and training yourself to speak from the Thorax means you are speaking from your emotions. Which means you are speaking the truth – speaking from the heart. Such speakers are usually eloquent.

The Costal Diaphragm is a fresh start for those who stutter. Not only is there a fresh breathing muscle, there is a fresh breathing nerve – the C3 root and the left branch of the Phrenic nerve.

The ribs, inter-costal muscles, alveoli, abdominus rectus, abdominal obliques, and elastic fibers in the lungs

If you want to know every little detail about the physiological mechanics of inhalation and exhalation, you're in for some work as it is an incredibly complex process. For those who insist on understanding before taking one step further, here is an overview. The rest you can find in any medical book on the respiratory system, although it is doubtful you'll find much on the separate functioning of the Crural and Costal parts of the Diaphragm without getting into very specialized readings.

Your ribs act like a bucket handle. Or a pump handle. Their hinges are on the vertebrae. There are many muscles controlling the movement of the ribs including the Costal Diaphragm, Sternocleidomastoids, Scapular Elevators, Anterior Serrati, Erectus muscles of the spine. The main muscles, however, for rib movement are the Interior and Exterior Inter-costal muscles. These are very short but stretchable muscles connecting the ribs to each other. When the Costal Diaphragm and the Exterior Inter-costal muscles contract during inhalation, it pulls your ribs up and therefore out. Another set of muscles, the Parasternal Inter-cartilaginous, also lift the front of the ribs. The Interior Inter-costal muscles are still relaxed, but get stretched. This increases the area of the Thorax and helps to create the vacuum. When the Costal Diaphragm and Inter-costal muscles relax during normal exhalation, the ribs return (down and in) to their resting position.

In normal exhalation, the main force of outward airflow is elastic recoil from the little air sacks in the lungs called alveoli. There is also an elastic recoil from other tissues such as elastic fibers in the lung and the pleural membrane. If inhalation was from the Costal Diaphragm/External Inter-costals, there is also elastic recoil from the internal Inter-costal muscles that have been stretched. The rate and smoothness of normal exhalation is controlled by the relaxation of the Crural and/or Costal Diaphragm and, mainly, the Exterior Inter-costals.

Now, if more forced exhalation of air is required, say, for shouting, tuba playing, blowing up balloons etc., the Interior Inter-costals contract to make the ribs collapse faster. Then here comes the big abdominal muscle along with his buddies the External and Internal Obliques, and Transversus Abdominis. These contract to make the abdomen smaller thereby forcing the top of the Diaphragm faster up into the Thorax. This apparently functions by way of releasing vacuum pressure in the abdomen and by literally pushing the abdominal contents up against the domes of the Diaphragm lobes. The Rectus Abdominis also helps to collapse the rib cage by pulling downward on it.

The theory

So now that we sort of have the physical idea of stuttering in relation to respiratory physiology, let's put it into a usable theory:

The Diaphragm (probably the Crural Diaphragm) in 'those who stutter' is chronically contracting and/or freezing when it should be relaxing, which disrupts the airflow (lowering what is known as 'subglottic pressure') that is necessary to create sounds using the vocal cords and articulators (mainly lips, tongue and teeth). One or more of these structures freezes, struggles and/or distorts (FSD) resulting in the stuttering block. If no answer is found, gimmicks (aka 'tricks' including leg slapping, using filler words, etc.) and word substitution are used. This will be elaborated upon below.

Different muscles are involved in different types of inhalation, and these determine which respiratory muscles are involved in expiration and therefore speaking. By inhaling (mainly) from the Costal Diaphragm and Exterior Inter-costal muscles, we allow the Costal Diaphragm to be the Diaphragm of expiration during speaking.

The Costal Diaphragm, with its separate enervation is not conditioned to contract uncontrollably during speaking. Therefore, using the Costal Diaphragm counteracts the freezing that leads to the struggle, distortion, tricks and avoidances we associate with 'Blocking'.

And to restate the second premise: to use the Costal Diaphragm and Interior Inter-costal muscles as the primary muscles of exhalation, it is necessary to use the Costal Diaphragm and Exterior Inter-costal muscles as the primary muscles of inspiration. The muscles of inspiration determine which muscles of expiration are used.

The physical cycle of blocking

Going back to the **Cycle of Panic** where the fear of being seen as someone who stutters leads to blocking, guilt/shame/self-hate, avoidance mechanisms then more fear and panic, let's look more closely at the physical dynamics of this thing called 'blocking':

Our belief is that the Diaphragm is the main physical reason or epicenter of the stuttering block. But there are other structures involved, mainly the vocal cords and articulators, which have also become, to varying degrees, dysfunctional in stuttering speech. After some observations, it appears to happen according to the following cycle:

1. The Crural Diaphragm contracts in response to fear, resulting in reduced or stopped airflow.
2. This in turn lowers the pressure below the vocal cords (subglottic pressure) to the point where vocal cord vibration is no

longer possible as the pressure below the vocal cords needs to be higher than the atmospheric pressure in order to produce sound.

3. The vocal cords, probably in an automatic response to this reduced subglottic pressure, become tighter (closer together) to rebuild the pressure. This, over time, becomes chaotic.

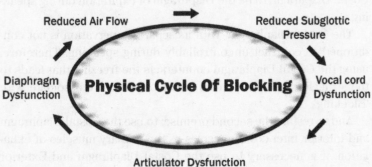

4. As our first concept of speaking has something to do with the lips and tongue (articulators), the habit of struggling and distorting these structures to get out our words becomes habitual and uncontrollable. We have had no idea that perhaps 50% of the physical problem is with the unseen/unfelt Diaphragm, and another 25% is with the also unseen/unfelt vocal cords, so most of our attention has been on our articulators that we can see and feel. As a developing young stutterer, I remember thinking: 'It's got to be something wrong with my mouth 'cause that's what makes the words ... so if I can just control my mouth I SHOULD be able to ...'. Over-control is as bad, if not worse, than under-control.

CHAPTER THREE:

Developing a new speaking technique

'If not you, who? If not now, when?'
ANON

Although we say 'getting good at the sport of speaking', when you decide you are really going to do something about your stutter it's better to look at this as a war of rebellion against a cruel oppressor. Out of control stuttering is not, nor will it ever be, your friend. It has and always will be your tyrannical enemy. 'Turn the other cheek' is something that will keep you oppressed. Once you've won enough battles that you start to 'believe' and feel confident that you have basically won this war, you can start looking at it as a competitive sport against a (sometimes) worthy opponent. But until then, this needs to be your number one priority.

This established, let's look at the physical and psychological weapons this enemy has been using against you:

The physical weapons of the enemy: freezing, struggle, distortion, tricks and avoidance

Observing those first coming into the McGuire Programme and my own occasional blocks, it's obvious that everything starts with breathing, therefore the Diaphragm that is contracting when it needs to relax to create the airflow that creates sounds and words is essentially freezing. Then we begin to struggle with the vocal cords (mostly on vowels) and articulators, thinking, especially as stuttering youngsters, that it is these structures causing the problem. As the struggle continues, our face distorts as we try to get our articulators (again, lips/tongue/teeth) to get the damn word out. And, although we can only hear it, there's probably some distortion happening in our vocal cords as well. Or else all these structures are simply freezing with no outward sign of struggle and no distortion ... while we're just waiting and praying the log jam breaks free before we pass out.

If no resolution is forthcoming for the freezing, struggle, distortion, what do we do? Tricks and/or avoidance of course! Slap that leg, bite that tongue, use 'ah' and 'actually' 20 times, pretend to cough or sneeze, or whatever else has proved at least once to break the word free. Or how about totally avoiding that word from hell and substituting it with something easier to say? Even your own name can be changed. No law against it, right? OR! HOW ABOUT COMBINING A BUNCH OF TRICKS WITH WORD SUBSTITUTION??!! Wow. Great idea. Might even work a few times to keep your poor listener from realizing you're a stutterer. Your listener will probably think you're a few sandwiches short of a picnic, but, thank heaven, won't see you as a stutterer.

Very good covert stutterers will totally bypass the FSD and go directly to (more subtle) tricks and avoiding. True communication is sacrificed for the façade of normal fluency. The listener can't identify the nervous shiftiness as stuttering, but is uncomfortable and feels 'don't know what it is, but something is very wrong here'. Life in the minefield.

In a nutshell: we freeze, struggle, and/or distort our Diaphragm, vocal cords and articulators. Then, if no solution is found, we start using tricks and avoiding, FSDTA for short. These are the physical weapons of the enemy.

Although it's difficult to say which comes first, our enemy has psychological weapons to use against us as well:

The psychological weapons of the enemy: Fear, Shame, Guilt, Self-hate, Sense of isolation, Panic

Fear of stuttering or being seen as a stutterer. Fear of being disrespected, rejected, etc.

Shame that you couldn't control the blocking, that your tricks and avoiding weren't working, especially after having been fluent before, and especially if your FSDTA was out of control in front of friends and family.

Guilt that you could speak better, or make your tricks and avoidances work better. Guilt that you were fluent yesterday (or whenever), but can't get a word out today.

Self hate as a result of the shame and guilt.

Sense of isolation: Going back to when you were a kid feeling very alone, that you're the only one on the planet with this problem especially when being forced to read aloud in class. No one to stand by your side while getting teased and bullied.

Panic: One can argue that anytime you FSD and/or use a trick and avoid, you're in a state of panic. Some would say we have the best physical and mental approach to solving the problem of stuttering ... but nothing will work if you're in a panic state. I personally believe that it is the sense of isolation that turns the fear into panic. But these all have to do more with psychology, which we'll get into in the next chapter. For now, we will deal with the physical, starting with:

Preparation

So, here we go. First some preparation. Like any serious athlete or musician (or soldier preparing for combat), you will need to:

Take Ownership: Be very clear that your stutter is YOUR problem. You own it. Not your parents, not your boss, not your wife or husband, not the author of this book, but YOU. And it is YOUR responsibility to do something about it. So:

Make a Commitment: Commitment means giving it your best shot. Do your best. If it doesn't work you can always try something else (and give that your honest best shot). But if you're going to do this, then do it. Specifically, make a commitment to:

- *Follow our directions* for at least six months.
- *Give up your old tricks and avoidance mechanisms* that got you by before. These have nothing to do with good speaking technique and will impede your progress. More than that, tricks and avoidance will increase your fear making even the best techniques ineffective.
- *Change your speaking personality.* I was told by one fine old gentleman who had conquered his own stutter that to overcome stuttering one must 'totally and permanently change one's speaking personality.' But when you change your speaking personality you are, when you think about it, changing your whole personality as most of how other people experience us is from what we say and how we say it.
- *Work hard* to develop the new physical and mental habits. If you come to this already with a good work ethic, great. If not, then it's time you developed a good work ethic. If you have a laziness problem, it's time to stop being lazy.
- *Develop discipline.* There are things that you will have to do which you won't necessarily want to do because of whatever combination of excuses you can find. You will need discipline to do what you don't want (but need) to do to reach your goal. If you don't have the personal skill of self-discipline, then resolve to develop it.
- Be courageous. Just starting this journey takes courage. You are, or should be, throwing down the gauntlet against your old stutter. As the old saying goes:

'When you draw your sword on the King, throw away the scabbard'.

You will need courage to keep from using tricks and avoiding words and situations. You will need courage to attack those fears, which have ruled your life and held you back. You will need courage to change. Most of us are not born with courage, but we can develop courage with hard work.

- *Persevere.* This war might take a long time before you win enough battles so it becomes a sport. Hard work and courage for only a few days or weeks is not enough. Be prepared to persevere however long it takes, then to put time and effort into consolidating your new speaking.

- *Accept yourself as a 'beginner'.* You have turned and faced this enemy called stuttering, making the commitment *really* to do something about it. You are, in every sense, starting to learn to speak all over again. In sports and music, you would call yourself a 'beginner'. Not intermediate, not advanced, not expert, but beginner. If you try to portray yourself as 'normal' (or advanced/expert) right away, you're heading for trouble. Accept the 'beginner' stage.

Your physical weapons

(To counter the physical weapons of stuttering)
Now that we are prepared to take serious action, let's summarize: The physical/behavioral weapons being used against us are Freezing, Struggle and Distortion, of the Diaphragm, Articulators and Vocal Cords. If no answer is found, we are compelled to use behaviors of Tricks and Avoidance. This leads to stuttering's Psychological warfare of Fear, Shame, Guilt, Self-hate, the Sense of Isolation, and Panic.

To counter the **physical weapons** being used against us, we have 4 MAIN **physical** weapons. These 'Big 4' are:

- **Costal Breathing**
- **Hit and Hold**
- **Block Release**
- **Deep and Breathy Tone**

Later in this chapter you will be introduced to other weapons, but these are the first ones to learn and master.

Your first physical weapon against the enemy: Costal Breathing (using the costal diaphragm to create the flow of air necessary to speak)

You will recall from the last chapter our theory that your Crural Diaphragm has the nasty habit of reacting to the fear and panic by contracting, thereby shutting off the flow of air over the vocal cords and articulators. No airflow, no speech.

Well, we could spend the next thousand or so years retraining your Crural Diaphragm not to react to the fear. But we won't. We're going to take the fast track and go to that new part of the Diaphragm, a new nerve root (C3) and a different branch of the Phrenic nerve. We are going to learn to breathe from the COSTAL DIAPHRAGM.

> *He who has begun has half done.*
> *Dare to be wise; begin!*
> HORACE (65–8 B.C)

This will require some hard work and perseverance, so **do your best**.

Stand up straight. Would be good to have a full-length mirror.

- Get a belt. Put it around your chest above the mid-point. Make sure it is tight enough to stay in place after you exhale, but not so tight that it causes pain.
- Take a full inhalation through your mouth by expanding your ribs. This should be fast, but not so fast that it is shallow and noisy.
- Make sure you have maximum rib expansion and maximum inhalation. Feel the pressure on the belt. Make sure you are breathing only from the ribs/Thorax (Costal Diaphragm), and not the abdomen (Crural Diaphragm).
- Without stopping after the inhale, exhale ALL your air moderately slow (again through your mouth). Feel the pressure of the belt around your chest release.
- Make sure both inhalations and exhalations are smooth and continuous even though inhalation might be faster than exhalation. Be aware of becoming too noisy.
- Pause for a minimum of five seconds before you inhale again.

Repeat this pause, inhale/expand, exhale, pause, fifty times. Really pay attention that you have it right as it is the foundation for everything else. Look in the mirror to make sure that:

- Your shoulders are down and relaxed especially during the inhale.
- Your face and neck are relaxed.
- Your head is still.

- Your mouth and throat are open just enough to inhale/exhale quietly.

You may feel tingly and light headed. Don't worry. You are hyperventilating. Just make your pauses longer after the exhale.

You can sit now, but keep your hands on your knees, your feet flat on the ground, and your back straight, preferably away from the back of the chair. Remember that it is not good to sit for too long (bad for your circulation), so alternate standing and sitting.

After about 50 to 100 of these *'Costal Breaths'*, one right after the other (remember to pause), **you must commit to breathing in this manner, taking a Costal Breath at least twice a minute during your waking hours** except while eating. Probably for the rest of your life. Just remember that people's breathing is generally too shallow, so developing the habit of deep Costal Breathing will be good for your health and will relieve a lot of stress.

Caution #1: Do not take these full Costal breaths while eating because you risk choking.

Caution #2: Because you are now doing much of your breathing through your mouth, especially at first when you are learning to Costal Breathe you must drink more fluids to keep your vocal cords from drying.

Caution #3: (Nose versus mouth breathing.) Although it is important to feel what it is to inhale and exhale through the mouth while you take a fast and full Costal breath, and to drill this way of breathing intensely until it becomes an automatic HABIT, you need to be aware that the nose is an important filtration system. Therefore, after the first week, make sure that you:

1. Inhale through the nose when you are not speaking.
2. Inhale though the mouth when you are about to speak and are speaking, as this is necessary to keep down the inhalation noise and to allow more air more quickly.
3. You can choose yourself whether to release residual air through the mouth or nose. Sometimes it is better to release residual air through the nose because then you are not breathing in the listener's face and it lessens the drying effect of releasing through the mouth. But, again, it can become a noisy distraction if too fast.

Your second physical weapon: Hit and Hold

For some talented people, speaking using Costal Breathing is enough to reach and hold onto that 100% confidence (0% fear) stage. For the rest of us mortals, we will tend to fall back on the old habits when hit by the fear of stuttering. 'Old habits' are, of course, the physical/behavioral weapons of our enemy: freezing, struggle and/or distortion, leading to the behavior(s) of tricks and avoidance. Because we've hopefully been using the Costal Diaphragm while speaking, this FSD is happening in the articulators and/or muscles controlling the vocal cords. From observation and personal experience, once FSD happens above the chest, it reverberates down to the Diaphragm so you have a 'full system shut down' (yes, even the Costal Diaphragm will freeze up when fear turns to panic).

So what is it about certain words and sounds that makes us so fearful of them? For many of us who stutter, it has been the first sound of the feared word. We generally have been afraid to vocalize or articulate this first sound fully because we're afraid of getting stuck – either stuck before we've gotten a sound out, or stuck in the middle of the sound so we can't go on to the next sound. Therefore we've avoided the first sound with soft contact or skipped over the first sound altogether. Or we've used various tricks. Or we've avoided the word completely. Whatever we have done, it has been distraction and avoidance behavior that has absolutely nothing to do with good, articulate speech.

Because we are afraid of approaching this first sound of the feared word, and because we are afraid of getting stuck in the sound, the principles of avoidance reduction say that we have to attack. We are afraid of the first sound, so we attack ('hit') the first sound. We are afraid of staying too long or getting stuck in the feared sound, so we purposefully stay in the first sound by 'holding' it out.

The idea is to **'Hit'** that very first sound of a word and **'Hold'** it out for a second or two without struggling or distorting. You have to be fairly aggressive to counteract the habit of holding back and avoiding. And you might have to hold it out longer and stick with it until you can release the sound smoothly. Remember to prolong the first sound and *not* the second (often a vowel).

When attempting this, be aware that all sounds in English,

(except the H) are either ARTICULATED (with lips, tongue and/or teeth), VOCALIZED (in the glottis with the vocal cords), or BOTH VOCALIZED AND ARTICULATED.

Before you read on, however, be aware that I did not come up with this from any book on elocution. This is all common sense stuff, as in not rocket science, that anyone can figure out by paying attention to what's going with lips, tongue, teeth and voice box on various sounds.

This understood, place your fingers on your voice box (aka glottis) so you can feel the vibrations. First, learn to Hit and Hold the plosive consonants, then the vowels, followed then by all the letters of the alphabet. If you feel vibration in your voice box, it's vocalized. If something is going on with your Articulators (lips, tongue and/or teeth), then it's Articulated. If there's vibration *and* something going on with your articulators, it's both. Roll up your sleeves, and start working on:

Plosive Consonants
We start with these because they usually cause we who stutter the most trouble. Remember, Hit and Hold *only* the first sound:

B as in 'Baker' (articulated and vocalized)
C (hard) as in 'Cattle' (only articulated) [same as K]
D as in 'Dixon' (articulated and vocalized)
G as in 'Gatwick' (articulated and vocalized)
K as in 'Kitchen' (same as hard C)
P as in 'Peter' (only articulated)
Q as in 'Quick' (same as hard C) Note – just the Q sound (as in K – not 'Kw')
T as in 'Table' (only articulated)

Remember you are saying all these sounds and words with a full, quiet Costal Breath, and making sure there is no pause or release of air after you fully inhale.

Vowels
If you were paying attention in basic English class, you know these as A, E, I, O, U and sometimes Y when pronounced as an I like in 'hydrant'. And there are a few exceptions like when O is pronounced

as W in 'one' or a U pronounced as a 'Y' in 'utilize'. All this understood, remember as you practice your Hit and Hold on words
beginning with vowels that true vowel sounds are ONLY vocalized,
not articulated.

H

H is just an audible exhalation of air. Because it is neither articulated nor vocalized, H is difficult to get hold of. The tendency is to
blow out all your air before going on to the next sound, which is
usually a vowel sound. There are two approaches to dealing with
the pesky H:

- Hit and Hold the second (vowel) sound as well as the breathy H
  sound. Keep at this until you don't feel the need to hit and hold
  (because your confidence is 100%). If, however, you're still getting hung up;
- Just hit and hold the second sound (vowel). Remember, this is
  the ONLY time you hit and hold the second sound. Keep at it
  until you can add that breathy H and don't feel the need to Hit
  and Hold.

The other sounds

Now that you've mastered the Hit and Hold on the plosive consonants, H and vowels and you can hear and feel whether they are
articulated, vocalized or both, we go on to the rest of the alphabet
most of which the elocution experts call 'soft consonants':

F ... 'Frank' only articulated

G ... (soft) 'Germany' articulated and vocalized

J ... 'Jerry' same as soft G

L ... 'Larry' articulated and vocalized

M ...'mother' articulated and vocalized

N ... 'Nancy' articulated and vocalized (note on M and N where
the air goes)

R ... 'Real' articulated and vocalized

S ... 'Stutter' only articulated (note the use of teeth as articulators)

V ... 'Virgil' articulated and vocalized

W ... 'Woman' articulated and vocalized

X ... 'Xylophone' articulated and vocalized (what articulators are being used?)

Y ... 'Youth' articulated and vocalized

Z ... 'Zebra' same as X

Incidentally, X-ray starts with an 'E' sound.

Some other things to be aware of: To really master the Hit and Hold, see what sounds have the same articulation the only difference being one is vocalized and the other is not. For example, B and P, D and T, S and Z, etc. Try yourself to figure out the others by adding vocalization to those that are only articulated. And there are so many others to get to know like different pronunciation for TH ('the' and 'thistle'), SH, CH, etc.

Your third physical weapon: Block Release

Now that you are an expert on how sounds are formed and have mastered these using Costal Breathing, here is another technique, 'weapon' if you will, to counteract FSD(TA) called the 'Block Release'. This is when you feel FSD starting to happen and you simply release your air, pause, take another Costal Breath and attack the sound/word again. This is a better alternative than going into a full blown FSD (or using tricks and avoiding) thereby making that which makes you feel bad stronger. Here are some things to think about when learning and practicing Block Release:

- Release the very first sound of whatever is starting to get you (FSD).
- Make sure you release all of your air, pause and take another full quiet Costal Breath before hitting it again.
- You can also mix in the Hit and Hold with Block Release.

Your fourth physical weapon: Deep and Breathy Tone

Since the foundation of the Programme in 1994, many of us have found that lowering our voice tone, besides being more eloquent, is a powerful weapon against FSD(TA). This goes for the ladies as well. So effective has this been that we've included it in our Big 4 weapons.

How? Just listen to your voice tone and keep trying to get it as deep as you can. You might want to use a piano and follow the notes down the keyboard until you reach the tone that is as deep as possible, yet reasonably comfortable.

Once you've gotten down deep enough, you need to add some air so that you're getting a breathy sound. The idea of it here is to keep the deep tone from turning 'guttural' thereby straining the vocal cords. By adding a bit of breathiness to the sound you are allowing the vocal cords to stay even more relaxed.

Now, drill all you've learned so far until it feels right. Just a few words per breath using the Costal Breath (CB), Hit and Hold (HH), Block Release (BR), and Deep and Breathy (DB). Then add more words, but try to limit to 5 words per breath. Here below is an illustration of the Basic Cycle of Speaking. Make sure you add in HH and BR.

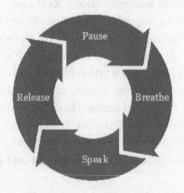

The basic cycle of speaking

More specifically:
- Pause for 2 to 5 seconds.
- Take a full, quiet reasonably fast Costal breath.
- Say your maximum five- word phrase making sure there is no gap between the inhale and delivery. In the beginning stage, make sure you practice the Big 4.
- Release all your air.
- Pause for another 2 to 5 seconds before repeating the phrase or saying a new phrase.

Other weapons to add to your arsenal

Once you've mastered the basic cycle of speech and the Big 4 major weapons against FSD(TA), here are other weapons to add to your arsenal, some of which you might want to include in your main arsenal. We've compiled these (including your Big 4) into the 'Checklist' you see below, with short explanations. After this you'll get some other techniques and concepts and the in-depth explanations.

The Checklist

Why the Checklist? So you can focus, thereby making each component stronger. Then the whole system gets stronger.

Why Exaggerate? Also makes each component, therefore the whole system, stronger, and ensures that they will hold up 'under fire' in real life situations.

Pause
- *Resist time pressure:* Speak when you're ready. Don't let yourself be rushed. You need to give yourself time to do (at least some of) what follows on this checklist. If you are rushing, you're panicking. Nothing works if you're in a state of panic.
- *Release residual air:* Make sure all the air in your lungs is released. In sports terms, it's the same as starting in the 'ready position'.
- *Center and Clarify:* For right now, this just means concentrate, and remember that you are someone working hard to overcome stuttering and become a good speaker.
- *Formulate:* Decide precisely the words you want to use, and hear them in your head before you actually speak.
- *Establish and maintain eye contact:* It's part of being a good speaker and is good for concentration. Looking away is like running away, and running away is avoidance, which increases the fear and leads to panic and blocking.

Inhale
- *Fast Costal breath:* Make sure your rib expansion and inhalation is fast enough to counteract holding back. BUT NOT SO FAST IT

BECOMES SHALLOW AND NOISY! Not too fast, not too slow. Find the right 'tempo'.

- *Full Costal breath:* Make sure your rib expansion and inhalation is full. You'll know by how the belt tightens on your chest. *(Think 'full, quiet, just fast enough')*
- *Quiet in the chest, face and neck relaxed, head still, shoulders down:* Keep your inhalation quiet by opening your mouth just wide enough to not make a whistling sound, and open your throat enough so it doesn't make a noise as it passes over your vocal cords. Monitor yourself to make sure your face stays relaxed, your head still and shoulders down.

Speak
- *Perfect timing:* Make sure there is no gap between the inhalation and the first sound of the first word. Do not release any air after the inhale. Make sure especially that you aren't throwing in one of those sneaky tricks to help you get out the word.
- *Assertive first sound:* This will counteract the tendency we who stutter have to hold back on those first sounds.
- *Deep and breathy tone:* Get your voice tone down deep as you can. Add some breathiness to take the strain off the vocal cords.
- *Keep moving forward, no holding back:* Once you're off to a good start, keep going until it's time to release your air and pause.
- *Articulate:* Give each word its proper pronunciation, enunciation, inflection, etc. Be concise and delete filler words.
- *Release residual air:* Back to the 'ready position'. Note that this important step is also at the top.

Additional things

Besides the Big 4, Basic Cycle, and the Checklist, you will need a few other concepts and techniques to get you going. Practice these like you would anything else:

Cancellation: There is a basic concept in psychology that the last thing we do before doing something is what gets reinforced (made stronger). We have had many years of reinforcing the old dysfunctional habit of speaking (FSDTA). Every time you let yourself get away with the old way of speaking, especially any kind of freezing, struggle, distortion or use of tricks or avoiding certain words or sounds, this becomes stronger. So make sure you pay attention, listen, voice-record, and, when possible watch yourself in a mirror or video. If it's not right, do it again.

Smooth, continuous Diaphragm movement: A good tennis stroke (or most any athletic motion) is, once begun, smooth and continuous. Trouble usually arises when there is any kind of stoppage of motion. Tennis coaches call this a 'hitch.' But it usually does not cause problems unless the player is under pressure. Why? Because tension (caused by the fear of losing) has a chance to get in and cause the muscles to tighten and sometimes freeze. This, mentioned in the first chapter, is called 'choking'.

Same thing with the Diaphragm. If you allow it to stop at some point during its motion, the fear will take over and cause it to contract when it needs to relax. Again, this will generally happen when the pressure is on.

Now, there are two problems: One is that, because the Diaphragm comes down before it goes up, there will always be a certain amount of stopping between the inhale and exhale, however small. Your job is to make this 'hitch' as short as possible. Again, the only time the Diaphragm perceptively stops moving is during the pause when your breath is out.

The other problem comes later when you are feeling a strong fluency but are not quite 'there.' As you become more spontaneous and automatic, you will tend to get sloppy with your Diaphragm motion. When you get sloppy, your Costal Diaphragm is no longer moving smoothly from up to down to up. Or you might even be speaking from the Crural Diaphragm. There are all kinds of little hitches and glitches that will soon become habitual. This is called normal speech. Unfortunately, it is destructive to you because your fear in certain situations is greater than for non-stutterers. These little hitches give the fear a chance to freeze your Diaphragm.

There will come a time when you can be sloppy, but not until you haven't blocked for several months. And when you do have a block (or series of) after a long period of fluency, you need to realize that it is primarily because your Diaphragm motion is no longer smooth. This means that you will need to get down and do some hard work to work out the hitches.

Perhaps a good thing to remember is 'a rolling stone gathers no moss.' A moving Diaphragm gathers no blocks.

The urge to be a totally normal speaker with normal bumbles, and stumbles, poor formulation, and unnecessary words will become quite overwhelming. Perhaps at first it will be like trying to keep a baby from being born. There is probably nothing that you or I or anyone can do to prevent it. However, after you've had your fling with normal speech, you would do well to continue your journey towards eloquent speech. A full, smooth from up-to-down-to-up Diaphragm motion produces eloquent speech just like a full, smooth tennis stroke produces a good shot. Why not keep your Diaphragm operating smoothly and fully and be an excellent speaker rather than a sloppy, normal speaker?

Monitor: Listen and look at yourself using voice recorders, mirrors, video cameras, Skype, and friends. Those little habits of your old way of speaking, including FSDTA, will try to come back. You will probably not even be aware of it happening and are probably feeling fear-free and 100% confident. Then you get 'ambushed' by the fear and find yourself freezing, struggling, distorting and possibly even using tricks and avoiding. This can be the start of a trip back to the swamp if you don't take action.

But you can stop this process by monitoring yourself using:

- *Voice record and/or Video* yourself during conversations. Most cell phones and computers have an audio recording function. Some have video functions as well which is even better because you can spot any old, trick-based mannerisms that might be creeping back.
- *Skype:* If you have a basic computer and internet, this is a great way to have free conversations with a lot of people around the world. Not only that, when you turn your video on, you can watch yourself as you speak. Those with iPhones have all kinds of video/audio apps to help you monitor yourself.
- *Friends and family:* One of the things you will have to do is be 'open and honest' about who you are and what you're doing.

Take this one step further, show them what to watch out for, and ask them to help you cancel.

Concentration: Getting out of your own way.
Tim Gallwey, in his book *The Inner Game of Tennis*, talks about your body already knowing exactly how to produce a good tennis stroke. One simply needs to get one's ego out of the way and concentrate fully on the ball. The book *Zen and the Art of Archery* talks about this too.

After you have spent enough time habituating the Big 4 and the checklist, concentration will allow all those complicated things to happen automatically. Concentration is a big part of Centering and Clarifying. When learning a skill, you must think about what you are doing and struggle at first. But later, thinking gets in your way.

Once you have retrained your Diaphragm, articulators and vocal cords, concentrating on almost anything, such as the reflection in your listener's eyes, the deepness of your voice or a spot on your thumb, allows your body to perform and co-ordinate all those functions necessary for speech. Concentration is a great tool for controlling fear and keeping it from turning into panic.

> *The art of medicine consists of amusing the patient*
> *while nature cures the disease.*
> VOLTAIRE

More explanations

Here are some more in-depth explanations. Keep in mind, however, that much understanding will come from simply taking action. If you don't fully understand despite these explanations, don't let it keep you from doing the required work.

> *Explaining metaphysics to the nation – I wish he would*
> *explain his explanation.*
> LORD BYRON (1788–1824)

Why the belt?
The idea is that you need to develop the habit of speaking from the Costal Diaphragm rather than the Crural Diaphragm. This means

learning to inhale using your ribs rather than your abdomen. Feeling the belt tighten on your chest lets you know that you are indeed using your ribs to inhale. It also gets your attention down in your chest where your voice is resonating rather than up in your vocal cords and articulators.

More about 'why the checklist?'
Funny thing about San Francisco's Golden Gate Bridge; it's constantly being painted. It takes so long to paint the thing that by the time the painters have finished, it is time to start over again. Same with your new speaking personality. You will find that while you are working on, say, formulation, your 'fast and full' will suffer. So you go back to fast and full and get that back in shape. And so forth. You keep at it until every part of the method is perfect and running smoothly as a whole system, and unlike the Golden Gate Bridge, you will come to the point where you can stop working on it. In this respect, it is more like sanding and polishing a rough piece of wood. Perhaps better is the process of writing and editing a book.

Musicians and athletes experience this. While a beginner piano player is focusing on his left hand, his right-hand performance falls apart. He keeps working on it until it is functioning perfectly and automatically. Then he can focus on experiencing the music.

A tennis player will do the same thing. While concentrating on getting his racket under the ball, his shoulder turn or footwork may fall apart. So he goes back and concentrates on these things for a while. Once his form is perfect and working together smoothly as a system, he can think about the strategy needed to win a match.

Why resist time pressure?
Ever notice a good tennis player before they serve? Good tennis players take a lot of time before they serve. They bounce the ball. They see what part of the service court they want to hit. They center themselves. If their ball toss is not perfect, they let it go and toss again. Good tennis players give themselves all the time they need to produce a good serve. They do not rush. Bad tennis players usually rush their serves and everything else.

The same thing with speaking. Those of us who stutter almost universally succumb to time pressure. We panic and rush, thinking the universe will come to an end if we don't respond immediately.

It is one of the many approach-avoidance conflicts. Desire to be quick enough versus fear of being too slow. It's probably the approach-avoidance conflict that started the whole stuttering process when you were developing your verbal skills.

By forcing yourself to pause before you speak you are resolving that conflict which has to do with time. For many of you it will be the first time you have ever given yourself time before you speak.

'Take your time' has probably been suggested to you before but hasn't helped. It probably made things worse because the fear increased during the pause. It was also giving you the message that there is something terribly wrong with stuttering. But now the game has changed. Before, you had no idea of the role of your Diaphragm in stuttering. All the time in the world will not help a tennis player produce a good serve if he does not have the basic serving technique. All the pausing in the world is not going to help you if your breathing technique is wrong.

The other thing about the resisting time pressure is dignity. Before, anyone could make you rush. Someone rushing is not dignified. So hold your dignity while you pause. Let the other people rush, and be undignified when they speak.

Resisting time pressure is like all the rest – you have to practice it if you expect it to hold up during the big game.

Why release residual air?
Even though you've started using the Costal Diaphragm to control the air flow we use for speaking, it can still freeze (and probably struggle and distort). To make sure it is used properly, you have to make sure it moves up and down in its full range of motion. Same with the ribs. Freezing is the natural response to fear, the solution of which is *movement* . . . and as much movement as possible of the ribs and Costal Diaphragm.

In tennis, it is like returning to the 'ready' position after hitting a ground-stroke or volley. Or returning to a deep knee bend after making a turn in skiing. Releasing residual air allows you to be 'ready' for maximum movement the next speaking phrase.

If you don't release, you will get into a pattern of taking shorter and shorter breaths. This can develop into yet another trick just to get the word out. The result is you're gasping for air before a feared word – playing not to lose, rather than playing to win.

You're probably also not resisting time pressure as it takes more time to release your residual air, pause, and take a full (quiet) Costal Breath.

Why center and clarify?

This is about knowing where you're coming from before you speak. Who are you? What do you want from these words you are about to speak? Is what you're about to say the whole truth? Is it honorable? Are you trying to impress the listener(s)? What are you feeling? If you do not know 'where' your words are coming from, you risk another approach-avoidance conflict.

One of the most important tasks during centering is deciding what role you will assume going into a situation. You will either be someone trying to overcome a stutter or a confident, articulate (maybe eloquent) speaker, depending on how you have been doing in practice and other situations. If your fear level is high and you have been blocking (FSD) frequently and/or using tricks and avoiding (TA) words, then the role you should assume is that of someone trying to overcome a stutter. If, however, you have proved to yourself that you can stay articulate even when feeling fear, you can go ahead and assume the role of a fluent speaker while being willing and comfortable with going back to the role of someone trying to overcome a stutter should things get out of control.

Centering has a lot to do with reaching the emotional and self-actualization goals. Failure to make progress in this area will prevent you from getting and holding eloquent speech. This is covered more in the chapter on centering and clarifying. In addition, you are encouraged to seek out the many resources – books and workshops – for personal growth.

Why formulate?

There is a very good chance that, between the fear and avoidance, you seldom or never really think about what you want to say before you say it. Most people would do well to think before they speak. Also, just because so many people advised you to do this doesn't mean it's something to be rejected.

In sports, you can call it 'visual imaging'. A tennis player sees the flight of the ball from strings to an exact spot in the opposite court BEFORE hitting the serve or groundstroke. Once technique becomes a habit, this helps the body to perform the action by programming what needs to be done.

In music you can call it 'auditory imaging'. When I was having trouble with my attacks and initial intonation, my trombone teacher would instruct me to 'hear', for example, a B flat, before taking a breath to actually play the note. Sure enough, the note came out cleanly (good attack) and in tune (good intonation). My breathing and 'chops' (lips) knew exactly what to do to produce a clean and accurate B flat.

Start with one word. Hear it with your air released. Take your full (quiet) Costal Breath. Say the word. Do this about 20 times. When you think you got it, add another word and another until you're up to, for now, the number of words you can handle comfortably.

At this point, you can start speaking without using the Hit and Hold and Block Release so much, but keep throwing these in now and again for practice. Remember that you need to 'hear' the HH and BR just as accurately as you would a normally articulated word.

Formulating your sentence or phrase before you say it also forces you to concentrate. Now, this does not mean that you are editing out the feared words. You can, like any good writer or speaker, edit out unnecessary words, especially those irritating filler words ('you know', 'I mean', 'ah', 'like', etc.), but editing out feared words will destroy your progress.

You may hear the argument that it is good to be spontaneous. Maybe so. Sometimes. But most times, being spontaneous is a good way to keep sticking foot in mouth. Especially in business.

> *If one does not know to which port one is sailing,*
> *no wind is favorable.*
> SENECA

Why eye contact?
Historically, those of us who stutter have poor eye contact. The reason is obvious – we can't bear to see the expression on the listener's face as we struggle to do what so many people take for granted. Poor eye contact is undignified, a sign of fear or lying, is

uncomfortable for our listener, and is not eloquent. Good eye contact is a sign of self-assurance, respect, honesty, and is more comfortable for the listener. Although you do not want to stare during your pause, you must establish eye contact before you begin to speak.

More important, poor eye contact is an act of avoidance. You are avoiding looking at what may be a disrespectful, pitiful, patronizing, etc. expression. Remember, do what you're afraid of doing. And by establishing that solid eye contact, you are starting to move forward, which is countering the tendency to 'hold back' that is the psychological foundation of stuttering.

For a while, you will need to exaggerate eye contact to make sure you will do it satisfactorily in a feared situation. Later you will expand this to seeing the reflection or pupil in your listener's eye.

> *Father told me that if I ever met a lady in a dress like yours, I must look her in the eye.*
> GEORGE BERNARD SHAW

Why full costal breath?
True, you don't really need a full breath of air to speak. But you do need a full Costal Diaphragm motion to overcome the tendency to freeze, struggle and distort in feared situations. A full inhale + rib expansion = full Costal Diaphragm motion.

In tennis groundstrokes, it is critically important to have a full shoulder turn in preparation to hit the ball. In this way, you can get maximum power and control with minimum effort and minimum unforced errors.

Why fast costal breath?
A slow inhalation/rib expansion might be good enough for safe, non-feared situations. But it won't hold up, generally, in tough pressure situations. If it is too slow, it can also be that you are already holding back and trying to avoid.

By keeping your Costal inhalation reasonably fast, you are countering the tendency to hold back. *But I need to caution you again not to make it so fast that you sacrifice fullness and start getting noisy.*

Why perfect timing?

When it's time to speak, it's time to speak. And when is this? It is *immediately* after the full inhale/rib expansion. Not after a short pause after the inhale/rib expansion. Not after little release of air. (Remember, your Diaphragm must move smoothly and continuously once it begins to move). Anything else is holding back making you more vulnerable to blocking.

When I was learning to give my old Bedford camper van (his name is Farkwar) a tune-up, I was amazed at the difference a small turn of the distributor made in his performance. Timing. He started easier, had more power, got better gas mileage, and didn't explode while the family was on vacation a thousand miles from home. Just the fourth gear went out, but would operate if I kept pressure on the gear-shift lever.

The point? If and when you have trouble (many blocks per day and starting to use tricks), it will sometimes be a timing problem. Let's consult with Farkwar's engine for an explanation:

> **Piston goes down and draws in a mixture of gas and air. Piston moves up compressing the fuel mixture. Distributor sends a high voltage current to the spark plug that ignites the mixture causing a small explosion. The piston is forced down. Exhaust is expelled on the up stroke.**
>
> **Now, the distributor has to be timed so that the spark reaches the fuel mixture at the exact right moment, which is when the piston is at the exact top of the stroke and ready to go down. Too soon or too late results in power loss, poor gas mileage and will eventually damage Farkwar's engine.**

Your speaking engine: Diaphragm contracts, then relaxes. It first moves down towards the abdomen, then up into the Thorax. A vacuum is first created in your Thorax, then released. Air is first drawn in, then expelled out. You inhale, then you exhale. You inhale, then you speak. Your words are like the spark in Farkwar's cylinders. Too soon or too late results in loss of power, weak elocution, and eventually FSD(TA).

The danger zone for you is between the inhale and the exhale.

That is where you are most likely to block because your Diaphragm must stop its downward motion before it starts moving upwards.

It must stop contracting before it starts relaxing. Unfortunately, it is impossible to have a completely smooth continuous Diaphragm motion. No matter how hard you try, there will always be a 'blip' (stop) between the inhale and exhale. HOWEVER, you can make this blip extremely short. Assuming everything else is also working properly, the shorter this blip/stop is and the quicker you begin to speak after the inhale/rib expansion, the less chance you have of blocking.

But to make the blip extremely short, you must observe and practice. Just make sure you are exhaling/speaking immediately after your inhale. And this is why God made voice recorders, video cameras, mirrors and friends.

Why deep and breathy?

Those who are successful with this feel their speaking process happening down in the chest rather than the mouth or glottis. Of course, some attention is needed in articulators and glottis when using Hit and Hold and Block Release, but you know by now that HH/BR are just tools to reach the goal of Articulate Eloquence. Deep and Breathy is (besides Costal Breathing) one of the 'Big 4' weapons that you use all the time. Besides being a great tool for getting that feeling of resonating and projecting through the chest, it contributes to Eloquence. Very few speakers with high pitched voices could be considered 'eloquent'. But beware that a too rich, strained, deep tone rasping from the glottis is not good for your vocal cords. So remember to add a bit of 'breathiness' to the deep tone. Recording yourself is a good way to do this.

Why assertive first sound?

There is a sport in Holland where one must jump fairly wide, not-so-clean canals. The jumper must run very fast, jump very hard grabbing a long pole that is loosely sticking upright in the canal. The jumper must climb the pole as his momentum makes the pole fall towards the far bank. If there is enough momentum and if the jumper climbs fast enough, the falling pole will drop the jumper on firm ground. If the jump and pole climbing was not hard and fast enough, the jumper ends up in the not-so-clean canal.

Why did I just tell you this story? Because the same thing must happen when you're facing a feared situation. You are trying to jump over (more like 'through') the fear. If the canal jumper jumps slowly and cautiously (holding back), he will get a cold, dirty bath. If you begin to speak in a feared situation with a slow and cautious (holding back) attitude, you will tend to freeze in the fear and get a cold, dirty block.

Another analogy is jumping through a wall of flame. Assuming you know it is only a wall and not a room of flame, how do you jump? Slow and cautious, or fast and hard? Fast and hard, of course, otherwise you'll get fried.

Stuttering, on the psychological level, is the act of holding back and avoiding while trying to speak. What is the opposite of this? Assertiveness, of course, and, in practice to overcome severe holding back, you should hit the first sound aggressively. Now, I'm not advocating becoming aggressive in your interpersonal relationships – although we will work on assertiveness later. What I'm talking about is aggressiveness in the breathing and mechanics of speaking.

Fast, full, assertiveness/aggressiveness will usually get you through that first barrier in feared situations. Once you are rolling, you will usually be fine. If not, it just means you need to practice more. And you do indeed need to practice it so that it is there when you need it. Do not expect it to work if you don't practice.

Remember: This fast, full, aggressive attack-kind-of-speaking is not supposed to sound natural. You don't need to do it in normal conversations except to practice. It is to counteract your habit of avoiding and holding back.

> *Don't be afraid to take a big step.*
> *You can't cross a chasm in two small jumps.*
> DAVID LLOYD GEORGE

Why articulate?
If you recall, the goal of the McGuire Programme is to become an 'articulate, eloquent speaker. There are many speakers who you could say are 'eloquent' but they aren't 'articulate'. This isn't good enough for us because poor articulation usually has a lot to do

with old tricks and avoidance. To articulate is to be very precise in the way we speak. This means to enunciate and pronounce the words and sounds properly. Many who stutter develop many gimmicks and fillers (tricks) to get words out. Sometimes they leave out sounds. Or substitute sounds. Or try to 'skate' over blocks by using soft contact. The final result is reinforcement of the avoidance behavior that perpetuates stuttering, and is anything but articulate and much less eloquent.

CHAPTER FOUR:

Dealing with the fear. Fighting fire with fire. Breaking the cycle of panic. Your psychological weapons

You now understand (from the previous chapters) at least our version of the psychology and physiology of stuttering. You should by now fully understand that Freezing, Struggle and Distortion (FSD) are the physical manifestations of the stuttering 'block' caused by approach avoidance conflicts. Hopefully by now you understand that if you don't find an answer to FSD, you start using your tricks and avoidances (TA). And you understand how Covert and Overt stutterers deal with FSDTA. If not, go back and read it again ☺. So, now, it's ALMOST time to take it to the real world.

> *It's all right to have butterflies in your stomach.*
> *Just get them to fly in formation.*
> Dr. Rob Gilbert

I said 'almost', because, if you recall, I also said our enemy has psychological/emotional weapons to use against us and that we would get into these in this chapter. During our intensive courses, BTW, we don't get into the psychological until the second day – the first day being dedicated for grooving the physical weapons. So it's now time for us to deal with the psychological/emotional.

You remember from the Psychological Weapons of Stuttering all that negativity set off by FSDTA? You know: fear, shame, guilt, self-hate, sense of isolation/being alone, and panic. Here are the Psychological Weapons we have to fight back with:

- **Deliberate Dysfluency**
- **Disclosures**
- **Overkill**
- **Support**

Fighting fire with fire. The main weapons against the fear, shame, self-hate, guilt, sense of isolation, panic

Most good athletes can deal with performance fear just with concentration, but, with few exceptions, we who stutter have some pretty traumatic experiences going around in our subconscious that make dealing with fear much more difficult. We have the habit of trying to hide who we are, and it is this hiding and deceiving that turns fear into panic and perpetuates the FSDTA.

So we who stutter sometimes need to do something extra to control and extinguish this fear. This 'something else' is repeatedly to do the very thing that frightens us the most. We need actively and assertively to show and tell people who we are and what we are doing.

In many respects, this is much like fighting forest fires where stuff like grass, brush and trees is the fuel that feeds the fires. Firefighters will create controlled fires called 'backfires' to burn up the fuel ahead of the main fire. No fuel, no fire. No fear, no panic. No panic, no FSD(TA).

Fear is indeed the fuel that feeds stuttering. Where we run into trouble is when we try to pretend we are totally normal speakers. This makes it very difficult to use any kind of good speaking technique, because, after all, 'normal' speakers don't have to use any techniques. Normal speakers just talk. No Costal breath, no pause, no deep and breathy tone, no release of residual air, etc. Just talk. It would be nice for us to be able to do this, but chances are you (as someone trying to overcome a stutter) need, like any good athlete, to focus on technique. But we're afraid to do this because then we will not be seen as perfect or at least 'normal'. So show some courage and come to terms with who you are and what you're doing.

How do we who stutter 'light a backfire' to burn the fuel that is fueling the panic and blocking (FSDTA)? It's already been said: SHOW OTHER PEOPLE WHO YOU ARE AND WHAT YOU ARE DOING! This is called 'Assertive Self-Acceptance' and the two ways of doing it are Deliberate Dysfluency and Disclosing.

> *We are healed of a suffering only*
> *by experiencing it to the full.*
> MARCEL PROUST

Your first psychological weapon: Deliberate dysfluency

And how do you show them? Simple. Just be very disciplined and mechanical practicing the Basic Cycle of Speaking, Block Release, Hit and Hold, using just a few words per breath, and whatever else you learned in the previous chapter. Exaggerate everything. And to take it one step further, by making your hit and holds a bit longer and by doing two or three block releases, you are giving the listener the heads up that you are a person working to overcome a stutter. But remember:

- To truly make this backfire to burn up the fear, you have to you feel confident enough with your speech to be less exaggerated, and/or you don't *need* to use a Block Release or Hit and Hold.
- To truly make this real 'Deliberate Dysfluency', you have to: 1) exaggerate your techniques, especially your Hit and Holds and Block Releases, when you don't need to *on words that are unfeared*; and, 2) have the actual mentality or thought going on of: *'I'm going to SHOW you I'm working to overcome a stutter'*. Otherwise you're just 'practicing' your weapons (which is good, too, but not as effective in reducing fear as having the right mentality).
- Those who have had traditional therapy might confuse this with a similar technique called 'Voluntary Stuttering'. There is a big difference. Voluntary Stuttering is done with the mentality of showing others you stutter, but not necessarily doing anything about it. With Deliberate Dysfluency used on the McGuire Programme, on the other hand, you are *not* accepting the freezing,

struggle, distortion, tricks and avoidance, but actively working to overcome stuttering and become an articulate, eloquent speaker.

- You are being 'proactive' rather than 'reactive'. You are attacking the fear of being seen as a stutterer rather than waiting for it to come to you. You are going after a difficult situation with the 'right' attitude, rather than waiting for it to come to you. Remember your 'assertive self-acceptance'.

- When you use Hit and Hold and/or Block Release to show that you are dealing with a stutter, it's important that you do this only on non-feared words. If used to counteract the FSD on feared words/sounds, it cannot be counted as 'pro-active' or deliberate. You're fighting the main fire, rather than lighting a backfire.

- When using the Hit and Hold, make sure it is long enough to let the other person know that you are indeed a person who stutters. Resist the temptation to pull out of it early. Exaggerate!

- Your deliberate Hit and Hold might turn into a real block, which means the non-feared word becomes a feared word. Then you'll have to get serious about a thing called 'Overkill' that we'll talk about in the next section. It also means that you have to do more Deliberate Dysfluency rather than less. Resist the urge to think: 'It's the Deliberate Dysfluency that caused me to block, so I'd better not try it anymore.'

Your second psychological weapon: Disclosures

This is simple: Just TELL THEM, openly and honestly, who you are and what you're doing and why. Get used to (and practice) saying something brief like: *'I'm working on my speech to overcome a stutter and have to concentrate on a few things.'* You might find yourself giving your listener a lesson about the psychology and physiology of stuttering, which is good for you (and them) too.

You gain strength, courage and confidence by every experience in which you really stop to look fear in the face. You are able to say to yourself, 'I lived through this horror. I can take the next thing that comes along.' You must do the thing you think you cannot do.
ELEANOR ROOSEVELT

Talking about your stutter and what you are doing about it not only reduces your stress and fear, it is courteous to you listener. I can remember Dr. Sheehan telling the story about how a person who stutters talking with a fluent speaker is like having a conversation with a baby hippo under the table. Neither wants to acknowledge the hippo and things become very uncomfortable. Once someone, especially the person who stutters, says 'hey, we got a baby hippo here under the table' ('I'm trying to overcome a stutter'), things lighten up. The listener, and thereby the stuttering person, is put at ease thereby reducing the stress. The less the stress, the less the fear, and the easier it is to concentrate. Less stress = less fear = better concentration = better speech. Remember, the big approach-avoidance conflict that we're all facing of 'fear of stuttering versus desire to be fluent', is more accurately the 'fear of being seen as a stutterer, versus desire to be seen as a normal speaker'.

Your third psychological weapon: overkill

We spend significant time on our intensive 3–4 day courses orienting new members to the concept and practice of 'Overkill'. On the Friday afternoon, they go out with veterans and watch them make a minimum 100 contacts with strangers on the street or in Malls and on the telephone. The next day, usually a Saturday, the new members (aka 'rookies') make at least 100 contacts with a strong veteran by their side. It all has to do with learning to 'Overkill'.

What is it? You will have certain sounds and words that trigger more fear than others, resulting in, you know, FSD(TA). You *must* attack these (thereby the fear/panic) with the weapons you've just learned. Not only attack but extinguish, kill, wipe out, etc. until you're bored with it ... Bored means 100% confident – 0% fear. But to get there, as mentioned before, you have to declare WAR and engage in *total* war.

Basic to war is the concept of 'overkill'. Too much is better than not enough. That is what Sherman was doing when he made his infamous 'march to the sea' during the American Civil War.

First do this on the phone, then face to face with strangers on the street.

Step 1. Get the yellow pages – either a hard copy or on your computer.

Step 2. Sit down by your telephone.

Step 3. Make your first or last name your feared word/sound (for me it was the word 'Dixon' as in Dixon's Electronic Shop in the UK). Or it could have been 'Dickson Davids' . . . or anything that is reasonably close sounding that can be the *stimulus that elicits the fear* (behavior psychology 101). Maybe your last name should be Pavlov should you have trouble with P?

Step 4. Dial a number. Hotels are best in the mornings, stores during the day and restaurants at night.

Step 5. Exaggerate all your weapons when asking your question. For example, when I was overkilling Dixon, I would say to hotels: 'David Dixon here, can you tell me the price of a single room for Tuesday?' For stores: 'David Dixon here, can you tell me what time you close today?' For restaurants: 'David Dixon here, what time does your restaurant open tomorrow?'

Step 6. Keep doing this until it's boring on the telephone. Be prepared to make hundreds of calls.

Step 7. Go to a busy street with lots of stores or a Mall. Starting with quiet stores, with a kind-looking counter person, ask a question that includes your feared word/sound. Keep going and challenge yourself to more difficult situations until whatever word was causing FSD(TA), is overkilled to the boring stage.

Some important things to consider when Overkilling:

• **Be aware that by taking a few, even one, feared word to the boring stage, other feared words will follow.**

• **There's a good chance you will have to repeat the overkilling process more than once on the same word/sound. In 2001, I had to overkill 'Dixon' to the boring stage 3 times with hundreds of contacts over 2 weeks before it was finally dead and gone.**

If you are trying to win this war on your own using this book, Overkilling will be difficult but not impossible. Just work harder, toughen up, show courage, and persevere.

Levels of overkill

To review and look at it from a slightly different angle, our 'enemy' is the fear and the FSDTA it elicits. But a better word than fear is PANIC . Fear of what? Panic from what? Well, fear of a sound or a series of symbols called letters that make up things called 'words'. Somewhere along the line, these silly symbols became super-charged with fear, probably because you got major stuck and experienced a great deal of the all too familiar shame, guilt and self-hate. Having rolled up your sleeves and made the commitment to put whatever time and energy it will take to Overkill, here are the stages, or 'levels' you will go through to reach the luxury of BORING:

Panic: Diaphragm, articulators and/or vocal cords are starting to freeze up. Fear is intense. Perhaps you're grabbing for those little tricks you use to get out a feared word or ways to avoid the word or ways to get out of the situation. Even in the easiest contacts with strangers, things are out of control every time. Out of 10 contacts, none feels right.

Barely manageable fear: You've stayed disciplined and have been pounding the word and it's starting to give. Still, out of every ten contacts there is freezing, struggle, distortion, maybe even using tricks and avoiding in one or more of the three areas of speech production more than five times.

Exciting fear stage: You're still at it and things are looking up. Like taking the lead against a tough sports opponent who still has the capacity to come back and thrash you. Out of ten contacts, you are keeping it down in the chest with no FSD(TA) more than five times.

Fun: Your 'opponent' is pretty much down and you have the game all but won, but it will come back if you let up. Out of a hundred contacts it gives you trouble only once or twice.

Boring: You've won. Out of 100 contacts, everything stays solidly down in your chest. Now you have to be concerned with staying reasonably disciplined and not sloppy. Boring is good. It is a luxury. It means that your confidence is 100%, your fear is 0%. Relish it, but don't get complacent.

Now go to the next word(s) that gave you trouble. Chances are any troublesome word(s) surrendered after watching you beat up his big brother, but just in case, do about 10 to 20 contacts to make sure he doesn't want to come out and fight.

And don't forget that the fear might, or probably will, counter-attack when you least expect it. Make sure you are prepared to put in the same time and effort to get it boring again as many times as needed.

Turn your 'perceptions' into 'beliefs'

Later in the book, you'll be introduced to the concept from John Harrison called 'The Hexagon'. In this you have two elements; Perceptions and Beliefs. Let's look at these briefly to help put Overkill into perspective.

A Perception is simply something you observe and experience. You 'think' it is true, or not true. Valid or not valid. You think/perceive that stopping eating bread will make you lose weight. Or you don't think/perceive that it will help you lose weight. Or you think/perceive that what we teach here will defeat your stutter ... or not.

A 'Belief' is simply a perception that has been proven true (or not true) enough times so that you KNOW it is true (or not true) as opposed to just 'thinking' it's true. You've seen the sun come up in the morning enough times that you KNOW it will come up tomorrow.

This is what happens when you Overkill enough times and take it all the way to 'boring' each time. Our enemy demands hard proof, solid evidence that you *can* defeat a feared word or sound. How many examples have you had to reinforce the perception and belief that you can *never* win against the fear? Thousands? So realize you're going to have to give yourself enough (probably not thousands of) examples of winning before the Perception of 'I think I can do it' turns into the Belief of 'I Know I can do it'.

Once you truly 'believe' that you can win this war because you have *proved* it enough times by winning these battles, this really becomes a sport where it is relatively easy to Overkill ... but you'll have to earn it.

What to do with a feared word

Especially in the early days, you'll probably run into a word or a sound that is particularly stubborn. You've done, say, 30 contacts and you still feel that FSD in those three areas. You might even panic enough to use tricks and avoid. Confidence is low, fear is high. You're Costal breathing and have tried all the major physical weapons/Big 4 (Costal Breathing, Block Release, Hit and Hold, Deep and Breathy) individually, or in various combinations. Here are some other things you can do to bring that fear down to a manageable level:

- *Use Deliberate Dysfluency* on the non-feared words before and even after the feared word.
- *Get some support.* You'll find that even a fluent speaking friend by your side doing contacts will be enough to bring down that fear (remember 'sense of isolation' to get you over the hump.
- *FIGHT past the Block/FSD.* Aka 'Prolong past the Block'. Only done on the phone with hotels, stores, restaurants, etc. Hang in there trying to use at least your Big 4 until, say, 5 seconds *past* the point where you could have said it with good articulation/vocalization. You'll probably be freezing, struggling even distorting while you *try* to use CB, BR, HH and DB. You cannot, of course, use tricks and/or avoid. Just tough it out. You'll find that after a certain amount of time, the fear/panic will subside. But you can't let yourself blurt it out! You have to wait that extra 5 or more seconds of HH/BR/DB using the Costal Breath. So what just happened? You went from reactive to proactive, and from real dysfluency (blocking/FSD) to Deliberate Dysfluency.
- *One minute hang-up drill:* Hopefully the previous strategy was enough to win the battle. Although rare, you might experience a word so fearful that even Fighting past the Block doesn't break it free. Time for, in military terms, heavy artillery and air strikes. The one-minute hang up drill is simply fighting past the block for at least one minute with the same rules: no tricks, no avoiding. You are actually trying to get the person to hang up on you. If they hang up on you, dial another number. You'll find that after 20 to 40 seconds, the fear is down so far, you *could* say the word fluently, but you have to keep going with CB/DB/HH/BR until the full minute is up. Then you go from mega-severe stuttering, to moderate-severe while you finish your question, then thank your listener profusely for their patience.

Once you've broken through the panic stage, keep going with your Overkilling. Keep your enemy, the fear, on the run until you can use any of the weapons or perfect articulation/vocalization without a sign of fear, much less panic. Keep reminding yourself, as you read on, that the object of all this is to break that approach-avoidance conflict, break the cycle of panic, and to eat up the fuel of fear that is keeping you from concentrating on good speaking technique.

Your fourth psychological weapon: Support

We believe that we have the absolute best physical and mental approach to win this war against stuttering, but we also know that the Sense of Isolation can be powerful and is probably what turns fear into panic. In the early days of the Programme, it became clear that even the best approach wouldn't work without support from other people who understand. That's why the McGuire Programme offers a lifetime membership and the opportunity to come back to as many Intensive Courses as needed, an International Phone and Skype List, Support Groups, and refresher days as needed. Members can also become Primary Coaches, Course Instructors, Staff Trainers or Regional Directors. For those of you trying to win this war on your own by following the directions in this book, it will be, as mentioned, more difficult but not impossible. Here are some things that will help:

- Tell your friends and family what you're trying to do, and that you will need help.
- Let them know that, at first, you will be a 'beginner' and will need to sound fairly mechanical for a while.
- Show them specifically what to watch out for (FSDTA), and the weapons against it.
- Ask them to help you Cancel anything that is not good technique.
- If possible, ask those closest to you to go with you out on the streets to watch you make Overkilling contacts.

A few more weapons and strategies to help you win the psychological battles

Concentration: Everything we're trying to teach you here requires concentration. Any athlete, musician, soldier, or anyone having to perform any skill under pressure knows this. If your thoughts are scattered so you have poor focus, your chance of achieving a reasonably high standard of excellence is not good. So practice concentrating throughout the day. If you find your mind wandering, bring it back. The ability to concentrate and focus can become a habit with hard work like anything else. Good concentration goes a long way towards not letting fear affect performance.

Replace the negative thoughts with positive: I recall my own tennis coach saying 'don't make your service toss until the thoughts of double faulting are out of your head'. He made me wait, similar to what you are doing in your pause. Then he said, 'repeat those things, silently to yourself, that you need to do to make a good serve'. The idea was by repeating the actual words: 'bend your knees, arch your back, spring up at the ball, etc.' there would be no room for 'better not double fault, what will those watching/my teammates/my friends think if I double fault this game away too, etc.'

Turbocharging 'hearing yourself': During your pause while reading out loud, make sure you've 'heard' the words in your head before they come out of your mouth. This includes 'hearing' the deep breathy tone. Practice this for at least a half hour, guiding yourself back every time your mind wanders. This may get boring, like most concentration exercises, but keep at it with the idea that you are developing your powers of concentration for when you are out there in the trenches of the real speaking world.

Visual focal point: Another technique taught by my tennis coach was 'see the seams on the ball' or the pieces of fuzzy felt during the ball toss for a serve or as the ball was coming over the net for a volley or groundstroke. Another thing was to see the line between the dark and light side as the sun hit the ball. By concentrating on this, you control the fear and keep it from turning into panic AND you get out of the way of your body that knows exactly what to do to hit a good shot.

Same with speaking. Practice reading, or just talking to yourself, while *concentrating* on looking at the small reflection of light in your own eyes in the mirror. If you don't have a mirror handy, a dot, piece of lint, etc. will be enough to practice. The smaller, the better. Make sure you keep whatever it is in focus as you speak. When it gets out of focus, bring it back into focus. This takes concentration. The more you practice it, the easier, and more effective it will become.

Auditory focal point: Read aloud or find something to say where you can focus on the process rather than content. As you speak, concentrate on hearing your voice coming out of your chest (not your mouth or throat because we want to get attention away from there so these muscles can do their job). When you're really in a tough speaking situation and the fear is high, feel it coming from your abdomen. Again, 'hear' the words in your head before you speak and 'hear' the words as they come from your chest or abdomen.

Visualization: A very good trombone player suggested visualizing the sound going out the window into our neighbor's yard. My tennis coach said to imagine the ball leaving the sweet spot of the strings and traveling, complete with spin and arch, to the exact spot I want it to go. Not only does that produce a better, more full sound on the trombone and greater accuracy and consistency on the tennis court, but the intense concentration required also displaces the fear and keeps it well away from panic. Trick is to do it during a performance or match. But, of course, it takes practice beforehand to make it work under pressure. Lots of practice.

Looking at the pictures of the Ribs and Diaphragm in the second chapter, try to imagine the ribcage, as a unit, moving up and out and the Diaphragm contracting downward while you inhale. Then the ribs moving, again as a unit, down and in, and the Diaphragm relaxing upwards as you exhale and/or speak. Takes a bit of practice and work, but you can do it.

Another simple thing to do, but one that requires the development of concentration, is visualize the written words before and as you say them.

If you'd like a simple computerized image of ribs and Diaphragm moving together, just drop an email to dave@mcguirepro-gramme.com and I'll show you where to find it on the net.

Mantra: When the pressure is on during a tough match, I have a little jingle (called in Zen circles a 'Mantra') to help keep away the double fault/easy 'shot blowing' demons. Before serving, my mantra is: bend your knees, arch your back, see the ball, snap your wrist up and across the ball, go for the (backhand, forehand, body)'. When returning serve, I'll say to myself 'see the ball, turn shoulders, see the ball hit the strings, go down the line/crosscourt'.

Same with speaking. Once you get the image of the Diaphragm and ribs moving together as you inhale and exhale, put it all to symbols (called words) with the following mantra:

'My ribs have just moved out and up, and the top of my Diaphragm contracted downwards as my Costal Diaphragm contracted, which created a vacuum in my Thorax, which sucked air into the alveoli of my lungs. But now, present tense, my ribs are moving down and in and my Costal Diaphragm is relaxing causing the top of the Diaphragm to relax upwards, which releases the vacuum in the Thorax causing air to pass over my vocal cords so I can speak.'

Repeat this several time while imaging the ribs and Diaphragm. Make sure the anatomy is synchronized with the words.

Tactile Focal Point: Feel your chest resonating as you speak. It helps to put your hand to your chest. Say something and concentrate on the vibration. Remember; give it enough time and concentrate.

Honesty and the four fears

We sometimes say to new students just finishing their first course: 'you have been cursed with fluency'. Usually, their speech is very strong and confidence is sky high after making 100 contacts and public speaking on the third day of the course. But we have constantly to caution them that there is some situation out there waiting to surprise them. Perhaps the sight of an important person at a party coming for an introduction. Or making a call and someone unexpected picks up the line. Any such surprise stimulus can unlock the great flood of fear still stored in the unconscious plus some new ones:

- **The old fear of stuttering.** Such chronic fear will not go away overnight. But it will go away after you have proved you can deal with it, and it does not mean a return to uncontrolled stuttering.
- **Fear of losing your articulate speech.** If one has been fluent for a long time, this is probably the greatest fear of all.
- **Fear of being perceived as a liar or foolish.** Especially if you have told others that you are 'cured.'
- **Fear of a repeat (and accompanying great disappointment) of relapse.** This applies to those who have achieved made significant progress, then and lost it in another Programme. The old 'here we go again' syndrome.

Just be aware that your taste of freedom from stuttering will increase the fear of losing it. Of these four fears, the most correctable is the one about having blown it by letting those around you think you are 'cured'. You'll have to go five years symptom-free before you can even think about 'cure'. In the meantime, enjoy your 'improving' articulate eloquence, and let everyone know that you're still 'work in progress'. ☺

Other things to reduce the stress and fear: Realize that this Costal breathing that you have committed to do at least once every two minutes during your non-eating waking hours will relieve much of the stress related to the fear of stuttering. So keep it up and even increase it.

To this, go to the book store or library and get some of the many books that will give you stress- relieving exercises. Find one you like, probably one is just as good as the other, and practice.

Taking it to the real world

You know what to do and hopefully have a reasonable idea of why you do this. And you've drilled it enough that the whole thing is comfortable. And you have a reasonably good handle on how to deal with the fear, which, just like the physical stuff, needs to be practiced and drilled.

Most of the time you were by yourself with a voice recorder and mirror, or maybe with a very trusted friend. It should be pretty comfortable. Now do two things:

* Write down a hierarchy of feared speaking situations, with the least feared (for example, talking to your cat), at the bottom, and the most feared (job interviews, cold call sales?) at the top. Be very specific.
* Start working your way up this list. But not too fast. It will not do you any good to destroy your confidence at this point. Just a baby step at a time. A good place to start is to call up trusted family and friends and tell them exactly what you're doing and openly and diligently practice your technique with them. Then go to calling hotels, say your name, and ask for a price of a single room. Or stores during the day, saying your name and asking what time they open in the morning. In the evenings, best to call restaurants to ask simple, quick questions like opening and closing time, etc.

Again. Drill. Drill. Drill. No soldier goes into combat with weapons skills half baked. No serious athlete goes into competition with a new technique that is half-baked.

CHAPTER FIVE:

Centering and clarifying

Minimizing the confusion that turns fear into panic. Self-actualizing. Reaching your potential

Verbal communication is using spoken words to convey something to a listener. But what are you conveying? Unless you can come up with something better, what you convey are feelings (emotions) and thoughts. These are the two main categories and both of these have to be clarified before you speak. And these two things are done either well in advance of speaking and/or during the speaking process itself during the pause. You know ... that thing on the checklist that comes after Resist Time Pressure and Release Residual Air.

He who knows others is wise.
He who knows himself is enlightened.
ANON

Eloquence and self-actualization

The goal of this Programme, as already stated, is Articulate Eloquence. We've shown you what to do to become articulate. Now let's get into Eloquence, starting with Self-Actualization. This is usually a lifelong process. The important thing is to be on the road to really knowing yourself, making yourself the most positive person you can be, and realizing your potential. Such a person seriously engaged in this process is full of interesting things to say. Being interested in what you are saying is part of being eloquent. Perhaps more important is that self-awareness – and becoming the best person you can be – is important to help you hold on to your fluency. Now centering, clarifying and self-actualization have to do with getting in touch with yourself – your real self – and presenting that real self to other people. Let me try to illustrate it with something from John Harrison, who wrote the Foreword to this book:

Self Actualisation

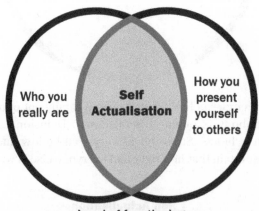

Level of functioning
Amount of Self Actualisation
How other people perceive you

The bigger the area of overlap, the greater the self-actualization, the higher the level of functioning, the lower the stress, etc. The reverse is true for a smaller area of overlap.

'What you see is what you get'. The illustration overleaf is an example of someone very much on the road to self-actualization. Stress is probably very low. If such a person stutters, it is probably very mild. If circles continue to overlap more, stuttering, even without the use of a technique, could very well disappear as it did with John Harrison. But, rest assured, it takes much WORK to get to this stage.

Self Actualisation

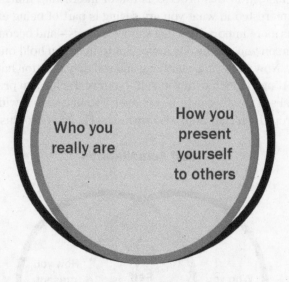

The two circles below are of a person totally out of touch with the fact nobody is buying his false self. Delusional. Probably belongs in a 'home'. Stress might very well be low due to being absolutely certain that he's right and everyone else is wrong.

Self Actualisation

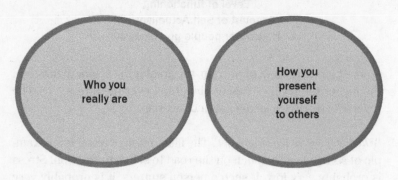

Man is the only creature who refuses to be what he is.
ALBERT CAMUS

At first this is simply knowing, experiencing and accepting your feelings and clarifying your thoughts before you turn all this into words. This is the road to self-actualization. It is one of the by-products of this journey.

The Hexagon

So how does one go about getting those circles together? John Harrison figured out that when all the components of oneself are functioning more in the positive than negative, fluency improves. He identified these components as intentions, behaviors, emotions, physical state, perceptions and beliefs. He then grouped them into what he calls the 'Hexagon' with all components connected by lines thus:

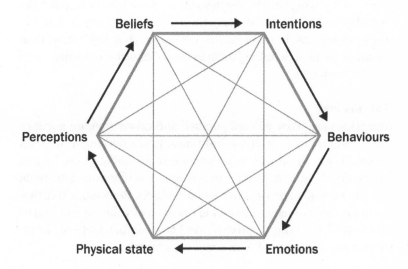

The Hexagon

Your Physical, Psychological and Social System (Harrison's Hexagon)

We, as living organisms, are a system comprising subsystems. There is a whole school of thought around systems as they apply to living organisms, including human sociology and psychology. It's called Systems Theory and can be quite complicated with concepts such as Entropy, Synthesis, Homeostasis etc., but, for now, Harrison's Hexagon is enough to get you going on systems.

If you look at the above model, you see the basic elements that make up your psychological, physical, and social being. And you notice that there are lines connecting each element to the others. So basic to Systems Theory is:

You can't change one part of the system without changing the whole system.

Notice there are arrows pointing clockwise. This is to show that the process of changing your hexagon from negative to positive starts with Intentions, then goes to Behaviors, then to Emotions and so forth.

So part of centering, clarifying, getting those circles overlapping and moving towards self-actualization – and probably the first step – is knowing your hexagon so you can see how everything fits together and so you can observe these components rather than 'be' the components. In other words, observing your fear rather than 'being' your fear. So taking them in the usual order of change, let's look at each one:

Intentions

Intentions are what you tell yourself and others you are going to do ... and mean it. And a lot of times, it has nothing to do with words. It has to do with what you are really going to do. I mean *really* do. What is important to remember is that your intentions have to do with approach-avoidance conflicts. Remember, too, that an approach-avoidance conflict in one area of your life will lead to the 'fear of stuttering' approach-avoidance conflict. Get your intentions clear ... make a decision and stick with it.

Behaviors

Well, maybe you have every intention in the world to do something. Or maybe you were just paying someone lip service. Whatever, your behaviors will say a lot about how sincere your professed intentions are. Ideally, your behaviors should always follow your intentions without a whole lot of procrastination. If this isn't happening you have an honor problem. You are not keeping your word to yourself and to others.

Emotions

There are all kinds of emotions, good and bad. I'd like to talk about the good ones, but they aren't usually what get us into trouble. Most of us have experienced a great increase in our fluency during the flush of love or excitement over something good that has happened or will happen to us. So let's talk about the not so gooduns like:

> **Anger:** Most of us know when we're mad. And expressing clear, righteous anger is one of the few times some of us who stutter have been totally fluent.
>
> One problem with this is when we're not sure what it is that got us angry. Then we're confused and it's here that we who stutter get in trouble with our speech because of the old: **Fear + Confusion = Panic.**
>
> Another problem with anger is that for some of us who have been brutalized because of our stutter, anger can quickly turn into rage. Rage is when you lose control and do and say destructive things that perhaps you regret later. Perhaps you are totally fluent when you are doing this damage, but the repercussions of destroyed relationships will later come back to cause you stress. And this stress will affect your speech.
>
> **Frustration:** Something you feel when things don't work out the way you want. The important thing here is to be aware of it, do some relaxation things to control it, and don't let it turn into anger. Confusion has a lot to do with frustration.
>
> **Fear:** for we who stutter, this is the biggie. The tendency has been for us to deny that fear and even run away from whatever is making us afraid. And sometimes, especially if you avoid it, that fear can turn into panic and terror. The idea is to admit you're afraid, feel where it is coming from (the general area of the Diaphragm), and be courageous in facing it. In the words of Susan Jeffers and the title of her book 'Feel the Fear and Do It Anyway'. Then of course the old Fear + Confusion = Panic kicks in. Part of this is accepting, too, that you have to deal with the fear.

Physical state

This has to do with your body. You know that usually 'more-trouble-than-it's-worth' thing that we never seem to keep proper care of. It's more significant than you think in terms of influencing the rest of your hexagon. For our purposes, we think of it as providing the energy to do things whether it be washing the dishes, going to work or cleaning up a feared word.

Think of how it was when you last felt sick or hung-over or jet-lagged, very tired and/or depressed. Chances are, your self-perception and belief in yourself weren't so good. And of course that didn't do your emotions, behaviors and intentions any good either. Then, naturally, you ran into major difficulties with your speech. Be aware that the two most vulnerable parts of your hexagon are Emotions and Physical State.

Perceptions

We talk about this in the section on Overkill. This is to do with how you experience things in the here and now. You can, for example, perceive someone suffering from the flu who walks by you without saying hello as having contempt for you, or as someone simply having a hard time for whatever reason. Whether you see the acquaintance as someone contemptuous towards you or suffering from some physical or emotional upset will depend many times on the rest of your hexagon. Perceptions are what you 'think' is true, and maybe you 'think' that you 'believe' it's true. You may perceive, after winning a few battles over your stutter, that you've won the war, but you're in for a disappointment because it hasn't really been proved enough times.

Beliefs

Beliefs are simply perceptions that have been proved true over time. You believe that these perceptions will *always* be true. You *know* rather than just *think* something is true. Your beliefs are the most powerful long-term influence on your hexagon. Your beliefs will be the last thing to really change you as you deal with the rest of your hexagon. Another thing about beliefs is that they can be passed on from generation to generation within a family. Negative beliefs (and perhaps some positive ones) always need to be challenged.

Another thing is how do you change your hexagon from negative to positive? Well, other than simply being aware of the hexagon and the process, you need to look at those arrows that start with intentions, then behaviors all the way around to 'beliefs'. Start with your intentions and make sure these intentions are backed up with your behavior. Here's a little tennis story to illustrate this:

The hexagon applied to a tennis match

If you start playing tennis, you will first have to drill the proper technique until it is automatic before you get into real competition. Once you start playing competitive matches, it will boil down to things like mental toughness, concentration under pressure, fighting spirit, persistence ... you know ... all those things that have to do with character. It also has to do with the hexagon. Here is an example:

I'd just played the first clay court team tournament of the season. I won my singles match against a much younger, higher ranked player. Surprised the hell out of me since I woke up feeling terrible from something I'd eaten the night before. So looking at my hexagon, I went into my match with my body (physical state) feeling terrible. And, boy, did that affect my:

- Emotions: Depressed.
- Perceptions: 'This is not going to be a good match.'
- Beliefs: 'No one can play a good match, much less win feeling like this.'

Important for my overcoming all these were my 'intentions' when I made up my mind that I was going to just do my best and see what happened. I forced myself to replace the negative perceptions and beliefs with positive ones and kept repeating all those things that I needed to do to play well – 'see the ball', 'turn the shoulders', 'move the feet', 'run for everything', 'fight for every point', 'close in after the drop shot' etc. – until it became a mantra not allowing negative thoughts to enter.

Now, also important is the fact that I had practiced hard all week with the intention that I was going to do my best to play well. I doubt that without this hard work put in to prepare myself that the positive thinking by itself could have overcome the effects of a body that felt miserable.

So the formula would go something like:

Positive, clear intentions + good preparation (practice and hard work) + persistence = more positive hexagon + improved performance + a good match + possible victory.

It is amazing how everything changed in the match. I soon perceived and believed that I could win; I was no longer feeling depressed and my body felt great. Looking at my opponent, he was pretty cocky at first since I was the oldest by far on the team (they call me 'the old man') and looked pretty tired, plus I'm still a bit fat. His perceptions were 'there's no way I can lose to this guy', his beliefs were 'I've always beaten old guys like this especially if they're a bit fat'; his emotions: cocky over his upcoming victory; intentions were to beat me, but to make it look easy as someone on his level is not supposed to have too much trouble with a tired, fat old man. And his behavior was to not concentrate as much as he should, and to over-hit the ball in an attempt to blow me away.

Towards the end of the second set (I had come from behind to win the first) you could almost see his hexagon changing. Because he couldn't blow me away, his intentions were in conflict (paralysis), he started making stupid mistakes, started thinking more about what his team-mates would think of him losing to the old man or even having the old man take him to three sets ... stopped believing in himself. He played increasingly badly and lost.

The hexagon, as stated, affects most all performance especially if you are under pressure. When you are speaking, you are, in a sense, performing – many times under pressure. Here are some points to remember:

- If your hexagon is more positive than negative, your performance will be better.
- If your hexagon is more negative than positive, your performance will be not as good.

• If your hexagon is in the positive, figure out what you did to get it there and what to do to hold on to it. Chances are things are going fine, but watch out for these things that we'll talk about more later:

Arrogance: 'I am so unbelievably good, (not to mention good looking and cool) I can't lose. Furthermore my opponent is a real turkey. I, on the other hand, am cool. Those who are cool always win over those who are not cool'.

Complacency: 'I got a great lead, just a few more points and I got him. There's no way I can lose. Therefore I don't have to really concentrate or fight for every point'.

If your hexagon is in the negative, look at your intentions first, make the commitment, then make sure your behavior follows the commitment. The rest of your hexagon will follow. You may not be perfect and you may block, but you will have given yourself the best possible chance to speak (perform) well. In getting your hexagon from negative to positive, pay attention to:

Denial: 'I really don't have to make a major change in my game to win; I'll win because magic is on my side'.

Intellectualization: 'Wanting to win a tennis match/speak well is for those who aren't secure in themselves, therefore I don't really have to try my best'.

Externalization: 'This guy has terrible technique and hits nothing but moon balls. I hate this kind of player ... he shouldn't even be on the same court with me.'

So make sure your intentions are clear and positive (even if you don't feel like it) if you want to keep your hexagon positive or quickly change it to the positive. Then make sure your behavior supports your intentions. Keep your promises to yourself and others. Doing what you say you will do is all about honor.

Assertiveness

You, if your stutter is out of control, have probably been a juicy target for manipulators. The main weapon of a manipulator is confusion. He or she will count on you: 1) being unsure you're being manipulated; 2) not knowing how to deal with the manipulation. You then get caught in one or more approach avoidance conflicts. And then your stuttering goes more out of control.

He that always gives way to others will end in having no
principles of his own.
AESOP

So why learn assertiveness? Six reasons:
1. Stuttering is the act of holding back when you speak. Assertiveness is the opposite of holding back. Moving forward (being assertive) in other areas of your life will help you to stop holding back while speaking.
2. Becoming more assertive will help you not to become confused when you run up against a manipulator (confusion + fear = panic).
3. Knowing how to be assertive will help you to stop your manipulation of others ... and will keep you out of the 'desire to be seen as honorable, fear of being seen as dishonorable' approach-avoidance conflict. It's all part of 'Centering and Clarifying.'
4. To be assertive with what you need to do to get good at speaking.
5. To help you be assertive with yourself, and stop manipulating yourself out of working hard and being brave.
6. Being assertive is one of the best ways to protect your emotions that, in turn, strengthens your whole hexagon.

I'm not going to try to teach you assertiveness here. Manuel Smith wrote an excellent book called 'When I Say No, I Feel Guilty' that you can get in almost any bookstore. He gives you a good description of what he calls your 'assertive rights' and teaches 'assertive skills' which are the tools to protect your rights and your boundaries.

But we do have a few things related to assertiveness and getting good at speaking:

Assertive rights of overcoming stuttering

In your suggested reading is *the* book on assertiveness by Manuel Smith called 'When I Say No, I Feel Guilty'. This is important for Centering and Clarifying. We have our own Assertive Rights specific to our war on stuttering that will eliminate any doubt and resolve any 'should I or shouldn't I' approach avoidance conflict. Mostly it is to help you deal with other people who may try to discourage you and manipulate you into not putting forth the necessary time and effort, but it can also help you *not* to manipulate yourself:

1. *I have the right to use my full technique.* Some people, especially in the early days, will try to manipulate you into thinking that the full technique is not good because it's not 'normal'. They might say something like, 'your stutter wasn't *that* bad', or 'you sounded better before'. And that 'manipulator' may very well be you.
2. *I have the right to really pause and take my time.* Other people, and/or you, might try to get you to think that you must hurry and it is wrong to keep them waiting.
3. *I have the right to take whatever time it takes for me to overcome stuttering and become an excellent speaker.* Other people, and/or you yourself, might try to convince you that you have a time limit to go beyond the mechanical stage. Some go faster than others. Take however long it takes as long as you're making reasonable progress.
4. *I have the right to be selfish and to concentrate on working on my speech.* You, or someone else, might try to get you to believe that other things are more important than working on getting good at speaking.
5. *I have the right to make contacts as long as I show consideration for my listener.* You, or someone else, might try to convince you that going up to strangers and calling strangers to work on your speech is wrong.
6. *I have the right to overcome my stutter and to become a strong speaker, which means making mistakes but learning from these.* You, or someone else, might try to get you to believe that being a stutterer is a bad thing. Or someone, including maybe you yourself, might try to convince you that it is wrong to want to overcome stuttering.

7. *I have the right to go for articulate, eloquent speech or to use Deliberate Dysfluency.* Someone, probably another stutterer, might try to get you to believe that going for Articulate Eloquence is wrong. Others might try to manipulate you into believing Deliberate Dysfluency is wrong. What you want to do, or need to do, is your choice and your right.

8. *I have the right not to care about other people's opinions and their judgments about what I'm trying to do to defeat my stutter.* You and/or someone else will try to convince you that not caring about other people's opinions about what you are doing to improve your speech is wrong.

Fallicies of logic: The manipulator's key weapons to create confusion and violate your Assertive Rights

Forewarned is forearmed. My mom sent me something years ago while I was in college called 'Fallacies of Logic'. It was, basically, a list of things a manipulator will do to twist things to manipulate others into thinking the manipulator is right and the other persons (including you) are wrong. Once this is done, they can get what they want, which is (usually) getting you to do what you don't want to do.

One of the effects upon your good self is that skillful use of fallacies of logic will confuse you. And confusion will lead to holding back – and holding back will lead to blocking as the all too familiar 'fear plus confusion = panic' sets in. Then of course, unless you are especially tough and assertive, the manipulator will get you to do what they want.

So the importance of reading further and learning this stuff is to be able to recognize when you are being jerked around by a manipulator. You might or might not want to confront the turkey, but at least you'll know what is going on, be able to keep your focus, and not be confused.

1. *Unqualified generalization:* No proof (facts).
2. *Hasty generalization:* Too few instances to support conclusion.
3. *Cause has no connection with effect.*
4. *Contradictory premises:* When the premises of an argument

contradict each other, there can be no argument (if there's an irresistible force, there can be no immovable object).

5. *Substitution of sympathy appeal in place of pertinent statements.*
6. *False analogy:* Different situations.
7. *Hypothesis contrary to fact:* Conclusions are not supportable by hypothesis.
8. *Poisoning the well:* Done by first speaker verbally attacking opponent.

To understand how these work, it is important to read through these dialogues contributed by Australian member Bill Fabian:

Bill tells his drinking buddy, Dave, a confirmed bachelor, that he's going to marry Kerrie.

Bill: 'I've finally made a decision. I'm going to marry Kerrie.'
Dave: 'Are you mad? Marriage is every man's downfall.'

Fallacy no.1: Unqualified generalisation: no proof, no facts. Dave has fixed ideas about marriage that he thinks apply to everyone.

Bill: 'What makes you say that?'
Dave: 'Some of the blokes in the pub who were married tell me things.'

Fallacy no. 2: Hasty generalisation: Too few instances to support conclusion. Dave only refers to the experiences of a few of his friends that he thinks will support his argument.

Bill: 'How do you mean?'
Dave: 'You know those alcoholics who are the first into the pub and the last out. All of them were married once and are now either divorced or separated. See where an unhappy marriage can lead you.'

Fallacy no. 3: Cause has no connection with effect. Dave implies that marriage leads to alcoholism, when the truth is that alcoholism is a physical addiction to a substance that often leads to divorce.

Bill: 'So you reckon their wives drove them to drink, eh?'

Dave: 'But worse still, my mates who are still married don't come down to the pub at all anymore. They're really under the thumb.'

Fallacy no. 4: Contradictory premises. (When the premises of an argument contradict each other, there can be no argument.) Dave assumes that because his mates aren't coming down to the pub that they are being controlled. The actual fact is that they probably have better things to do than go down to the pub.

Bill: 'I've got other things in life besides drinking at the pub, you know Dave.'

Dave: 'Well what about me? It won't be the same if my best friend gets married. I'll only have those damned alcoholics to drink with.'

Fallacy no. 5: Substitution of sympathy appeal in place of pertinent statements. Dave appeals to Dave's sense of loyalty to an old friend.

Bill: 'I'm sure I'll find time to meet up with you for a drink now and then.'

Dave: 'Look Bill. Remember that time you bought that pet dog for a companion. He chewed up your furniture and crapped on your carpet. He made your life so miserable that you couldn't stand him. It'll be the same thing having a wife around, doing things you don't like.'

Fallacy no. 6: False analogy: Different situations. Dave makes an illogical comparison between two types of live-in companions.

Bill: 'I think she's house trained, Dave.'

Dave: 'I can ask out any woman I want and you'll be going home to the same one every night. You must be some kind of masochist.'

Fallacy no. 7: Hypothesis contrary to fact: (Conclusion not supported by hypothesis.) Dave assumes his view of monogamy is shared by Bill and wrongly dismisses Bill's point of view as being one of self-hate.

Bill: 'That's true Dave. You do ask a lot of women out, but none of them ever says 'Yes'.'

Dave: 'Bill, I say this as a friend. I've known you for years. You always make wrong decisions. Marrying Kerrie will just confirm that you really are a pathetic loser.'

Fallacy no. 8: Poisoning the well: (Done by first speaker verbally attacking opponent.) Dave tries to give Bill doubts by ridiculing Bill's track record and attacking his credibility in making decisions.

Putting some time and effort into understanding these Fallacies of Logic would be well worth your time. As an exercise, take the above 8 examples, and apply these to your war on stuttering.

Centering and clarifying flow chart

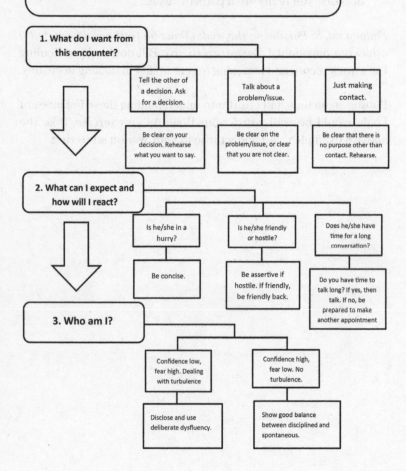

TOUGH SITUATION CENTERING AND CLARIFYING

Tough phone call or face-to-face encounter coming up? Do you just grab the phone or walk in and start blabbing? Not a good idea. Chances are you'll get ambushed with FSD or TA, and not make the best impression. Of course you've warmed up by being disciplined all day, made some extra contacts, etc., but now it's right before the encounter. Time to sit back for 3 to 5 minutes, breathe, close your eyes and center and clarify. Walk yourself through the following.

1. What do I want from this encounter?

- Tell the other of a decision. Ask for a decision.
  - Be clear on your decision. Rehearse what you want to say.
- Talk about a problem/issue.
  - Be clear on the problem/issue, or clear that you are not clear.
- Just making contact.
  - Be clear that there is no purpose other than contact. Rehearse.

2. What can I expect and how will I react?

- Is he/she in a hurry?
  - Be concise.
- Is he/she friendly or hostile?
  - Be assertive if hostile. If friendly, be friendly back.
- Does he/she have time for a long conversation?
  - Do you have time to talk long? If yes, then talk. If no, be prepared to make another appointment

3. Who am I?

- Confidence low, fear high. Dealing with turbulence
  - Disclose and use deliberate dysfluency.
- Confidence high, fear low. No turbulence.
  - Show good balance between disciplined and spontaneous.

Levels of progress towards articulate eloquence

Now that you have gotten everything you need to be the speaker and the person you want to be, here below is the big picture that will also help with Center and Clarify. If you follow the directions, work hard and be courageous, your progress from the swamp of out-of-control stammering, FSDTA, to Articulate Eloquence should be something like this:

Stairway to articulate eloquence

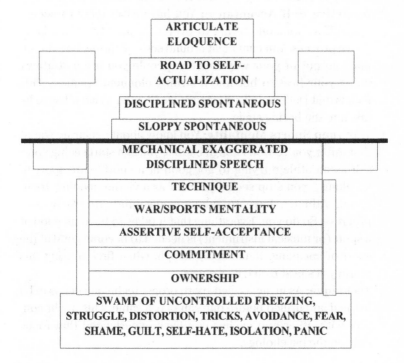

Explanation of the levels

Swamp: This is what brought you into the Programme. FSDTA is the in charge along with all the psychological garbage of Fear, Guilt, Shame, Self-hate, Isolation, and Panic.

Foundation: You want a strong platform on which to develop your articulate eloquence. As foundations are stronger when layered, this foundation comes in several levels:

- **Ownership:** Not only do you own your stutter (not someone else's problem), you own the responsibility to overcome it and become a strong speaker. No one else but you is going to do this. You own it and this is the first layer of your foundation.
- **Commitment:** Once you've taken ownership, you have to make a personal commitment to do something about it. It helps if you make this commitment to someone else as well.
- **Assertive Self-Acceptance:** You have assertively to accept yourself as someone trying to overcome a stutter. This is an active process. You cannot sit around self-accepting, but, rather, must go out of your way to show people you are a stutterer doing your best to become a strong, eloquent speaker. This means that Deliberate Dysfluency (see Chapter 4) itself has to be taken to the boring stage.
- **War, then Sports Mentality:** You know about declaring war at first. After you've won enough battles, you can start seeing yourself as an athlete trying to get good at a sport – the sport of speaking – you stop seeing yourself as a victim needing 'treatment'. Athletes have to take responsibility for their own progress. So do you. Everything that it takes to become good at a sport (or musical instrument) is needed to become good at the sport of speaking. Remember, though, when first starting this journey, it's best to see it as a war.
- **Technique:** As in any skilled sport, proper technique needs to be learned and drilled before one can play a game. This might conflict with other approaches you have experienced that focus only on the psychology.

Generally, if you're having more than your share of turbulence or chronically taking nosedives back into the swamp, one or more of your foundation layers is not solid.

Mechanical exaggerated disciplined speech: Until the technique is automatic and all feared words and situations are overkilled, you should be sounding fairly mechanical and not too many words per breath. This is a higher level of self-acceptance. You are being 'mechanical' because you are working to overcome a stutter and this is what you have to do to become a strong, eloquent speaker.

Sloppy spontaneous: You might reach that 100% confident, 0% fear orbit zone before you've really grooved your technique. You will feel so free and fluent that it will be very difficult for you to be disciplined and stay in the mechanical stage. It's much like trying to keep a baby from being born. You will use virtually no technique and will probably be quite 'normally dysfluent'. Congratulations! This means you have overkilled all your feared words and situations and are truly, albeit temporarily, free from stuttering and on your way to eloquence. You will no doubt, however, take a fall from here back down to the swamp. Then you will have to rebuild your foundation, stay longer in the mechanical stage and hopefully go to the stage called:

Disciplined spontaneous: This is where you don't really have to think about any technique (most of the time) for speaking because it is such a habit it is happening automatically. You have struck a nice balance between discipline and spontaneity. You are, by this point, quite articulate.

Road to self actualization: For most, self-actualization is a lifetime process. It is the process of overlapping your two circles so that what others see is what they get and you are realizing your potential to do with this precious life exactly what you want to be doing and know exactly who you are in relation to the world and other people. The important thing is to be on the road to self-actualization. This makes things you say very interesting to other people, and this leads to:

Articulate eloquence: You enjoy and feel what you are saying. Other people enjoy and feel what you are saying, and you hear them refer to you as 'articulate' and/or 'eloquent'. Beyond your wildest dreams?

PART TWO:

How to keep it

(The 'Directions')

To win the war against stuttering and get good at the sport of speaking you will have to DO YOUR BEST to WORK HARD, BE COURAGEOUS and PERSEVERE in following these 'basic' directions:

1. Breathe from the Costal Diaphragm all day long except when you're eating. This should be no less than two Costal breaths every minute.
2. Speak with at least the basic method whenever you speak.
3. Practice Hit and Hold and Block Release every day.
4. Cancel poor technique.
5. Overkill your feared words to the boring stage.
6. Keep pushing out your comfort zones by challenging your feared situations.

Even if you're on the right track, you'll get run over if you just sit there.
WILL ROGERS

CHAPTER SIX:

Practice

Practice is the best of all instructors.
PUBLILIUS SYRUS

Using the weapons

Now that you've been taught the major Big 4 and other weapons on the checklist, it's time to put it all together into an overall picture. There are 4 levels of uses of these weapons:

Reactive: Responding to an Ambush

Infantrymen on patrol in a combat zone have been trained how to respond to an ambush. Whether or not they survive will depend on luck and how well they can fall back on their training that has been drilled over and over. Hit the ground, find cover, return fire. The natural reaction is to panic, run, which greatly lessens chances of survival. Their drill sergeant reminds them frequently that it is not '*if*' they get ambushed, but '*when*'.

Same with your war on stuttering after you've reached the 100% confidence stage. Suddenly the fear jumps out at you and you start to panic, feeling the old FSD coming and the desire to use tricks and avoid. Not 'if', but 'when', because you *will* get ambushed. Whether or not you respond with FSDTA will depend on how well you have learned and drilled your weapons – especially Hit and Hold and Block Release. That's why you want to practice the Big 4 so they are fresh for when you are surprised by the fear – especially the Hit and Hold and Block Release.

Proactive: Practicing the weapons

Simply practicing your Weapons for the times you get ambushed is being Proactive so that when you're in Reactive Mode, you don't reinforce that which makes you feel bad and lose confidence (FSDTA).

Super proactive: Deliberate dysfluency

When you exaggerate and make obvious the use of your Weapons with the mentality of 'I'm going to *show* you I'm working to overcome a stutter' (aka: Deliberate Dysfluency), you are doing more than just practicing. Combine this with Disclosures (tell them who you are and what you're doing), and this will knock down the fear so that the tendency to panic is greatly reduced. Use this when confidence is low, and fear is high.

Heavy artillery/airstrikes: Fight past the block and the one minute hang-up drill

If you were an officer in a combat situation and your position was about to be overrun by the enemy, the last ditch desperate strategy would be to call in heavy artillery and/or airstrikes on your own position. The idea is that you and your men *know* its coming and where to take cover, but the enemy does not. You will probably have severe casualties, but there is a good chance the enemy casualties will be much worse.

This is similar to the Fighting Past the Block, and the One Minute Hang-up Drill we covered in Chapter 3. If you recall, it's when the fear turns every time to panic, you are back in the swamp and out of control. FPB and OMHD will knock down the fear and panic enough so you can concentrate on using your weapons.

More about developing habits

You have declared war on your stutter and we have given you physical and psychological weapons to fight with. Those who have had military experience, especially infantry boot camp, know that certain things have to be practiced (drilled) over and over so that when overwhelmed with the terror of combat a soldier will 'fall back on his training'. For example, the recruit will practice taking apart, cleaning, and reassembling his weapon until he can do it *quickly* blindfolded in preparation for that time the weapon jams at night while under attack. It must become an automatic *habit*.

For we who stutter, once we have survived and won enough battles to start 'believing' we can win and are winning this war, we can look at it more as a sport, albeit a serious one.

> *Bad habits are like a comfortable bed,*
> *easy to get into, but hard to get out of.*
> ANON

We introduced you to some basic physical and psychological weapons in Chapters 3 and 4. These 'basics' must become a habit. For these to become habits, you must practice.

You must practice at least enough to have a steady improvement. If you are not improving, you must increase your practice time until you show steady improvement. Defeating stuttering must become one of your life's top priorities. At first, it must take absolute first priority. If you have a busy schedule, you need to develop time-management skills. You might have to wake up earlier and go to bed later.

Tennis and Speaking habits

Looking at this as a skilled sport such as golf or skiing (or learning almost any musical instrument), tennis is not one of those sports you can just go out, pick up a racquet and expect to play well. Like in skiing where you have to train yourself to do unnatural things like putting all your weight on the downhill ski and leaning downhill (when your natural instincts are screaming to put your weight on both skis or the uphill ski and lean uphill), tennis requires you to do some things that aren't really natural and must be taught.

> *The harder I practice, the luckier I get.*
> GARY PLAYER (SOUTH AFRICAN PRO GOLFER)

For example: The natural tendency is to hit the ball flat like you would a baseball. Or to swat the ball using your wrist and arm like you would in racquetball. Someone, generally, has to teach you that you must get your racket under the ball to impart topspin and to lift the ball over the net and still have a degree of power. Someone also has to teach you to keep a firm wrist and turn your hips and shoulders so that you can torque energy that will produce controlled power.

Then we would also have to start talking about the why and what of grip changes between backhand, forehand, volley, and serve. Oh yes …then we would have to teach you about bending your knees and moving your feet. But wait a minute, then we have to get into how to hit an approach shot when you see that short ball not to mention the topspin lob, overhead smash, flat and spin serves, the slice backhand, down the line passing shot, sharp angled topspin winner, and, finally, the drop shot. BUT WAIT! Then what to do when your opponent hits you a drop shot?! I think that's about it.

Then all these techniques must be mastered and drilled until they become automatic if one wants to get good at the sport of tennis. Same with the sport of speaking.

How much is enough? The phone and the street

So you have put your head down and have given your word of honor to keep fighting until your stuttering monster is defeated. You have declared total war in this fight for freedom. You still have fear. The best places to start habituating your new technique, developing an assertive mentality and continuing to kill the fear are with strangers on the telephone or in the streets and shops. These situations are your 'war games' and practice matches.

These situations represent the lower part of your iceberg above the surface. There is no real consequence in dealing with strangers whom you will never see again. However, there is enough pressure involved to prepare you for the important tournaments.

The horrible hundred
Until your fear is 0%, and your confidence is 100% and you're starting to *believe* that you can win this war (and become an excellent speaker), your goal should be 100 face-to-face or phone-to-phone contacts with strangers *every day*. One hundred or more contacts a day will test your motivation. It is not easy. You will have to push

yourself, especially at the end, to reach it. One hundred or more contacts a day does not leave room to sit around intellectualizing and avoiding. You have to do it fairly fast, otherwise you will stay up past your bedtime.

For those of you who still think this is unreasonable and unfair, imagine yourself on a football team. The coach tells you to run laps after practice when you are already tired. You come to him saying 'Sorry coach, I'm just too tired to run twenty laps. It's unfair and unreasonable for you to demand this of us. Ten is enough for me now.'

Any good coach would not even argue. Their response would be: 'Clean out your locker and do not come back.' Period.

Good news and bad news: The bad news is that you have to keep doing 100 situations a day until you gain that 100% confidence where all words and situations are unfeared. The good news is that if you do 100 new contacts in addition to everything else, you will reach this freedom quickly.

Why quantity?

It has been argued that it is better to have fewer but longer contacts. Not necessarily true. Generally, anyone – even a stranger – willing to give you more than a few minutes will have patient ears. Your fear level soon drops. This is fine for habituating the technique and drilling points on the checklist, but it is doing almost nothing for habituating your non-avoidance and assertiveness.

We are what we repeatedly do.
Excellence, then, is not an act, but a habit.
ARISTOTLE

It has been initial contacts with strangers that have given you the most trouble in the past. You do not know if that new voice on the telephone or that new face in the street will be friendly or hostile. Understanding or contemptuous. Patient or irritable. You have thousands of examples of facing these situations with tricks and avoidance. You need at least several hundred of examples of facing these unknowns with dignity and assertiveness.

Good news and bad news: First the bad news. Strangers on the phone and in the street have generally given you the most trouble the past. You will, therefore, probably experience much fear at first. The good news is that, because you will never see these strangers again, these contacts will quickly become unfeared.

The Phone: Get the yellow pages. Sit down by your telephone. If you live in a low population area, you might want to get yellow pages from surrounding areas. You can find these easily on the internet. If you have a feared word needing overkilling, make up a first or last name of something that sounds similar. Perhaps it is the word 'direction.' Make up a name using that feared word. 'This is Dan Direction. Can you tell me the price of a single room for tonight? Yes, it is an unusual name. Thank you.'

We talked about this in the section on Overkill, but here it is again: The best places to call early in the morning are Hotels. Someone will always pick up the phone and not be angry at being bugged so early. Later on in the day, you can call shops. In the evening restaurants are good targets, but make sure you call back to cancel any reservations. In both shops and restaurants, it is best just to ask the opening or closing times. Again, the important thing is to get that feared word down in the chest with as many new voices as possible – this means many short contacts.

Get some newspapers. You will find the numbers of many waiting for you to call. They are trying to sell things. After first saying your name, ask them about the punctured waterbed, the comic books, the chain saw, the bicycle. Ask its condition. Ask if they will take a lower price for them and say you will call back. Call them back. Say your name again then say you are not interested. Thank them for their time.

If you run out of want-ads, restaurants and hotels in the evenings or holidays, you can call private numbers. Just be aware that you are bothering people in their own homes so, out of common courtesy, make it quick. Best to say your name and ask for the (feared word) pub, shop, office, etc. Your victim will quickly inform you that you have a wrong number. Just apologize, and go on to the next number.

Now, if you're especially stout-hearted, you can say something like: 'So-and-so (perhaps a feared word fictitious name) is my name. I've chosen your name out of the phone book at random because I'm trying to complete an assignment to help me overcome a stutter. Could I have a minute of your time?' They will either tell you where to shove it, or give you the time. The originator of this exercise (Heather Lucy) reports many delightful conversations with people who become very interested in stuttering and wanting to help.

The Street: Find a good-sized town or city. Go to the busiest streets. Go into the shops and go up to people in the street. Warm up by asking for things with Deliberate Dysfluency on non-feared words.

Then start using your feared words. Assuming you have feared word(s), ask for the (feared word) museum. The (feared word) pub. Try to avoid asking for an actual location – you do not have time to stand and listen to directions. And some sweet grandmother might lead you by the hand to a place you do not want to go. If you're asking for an actual place (store, pub, street, etc.), make sure you're going in that direction.

Disclosures are especially effective at knocking down the fear. You can say something like: 'Excuse me. I am a stutterer on a speech therapy course and my assignment is to tell a hundred people my name. I am (your name). Thank you for listening.' Of course, you should be using some Deliberate Dysfluency with this one.

Life is like playing a violin in public
and learning the instrument as one goes on
SAMUEL BUTLER

The 15-minute Sprint Drill: Back in my high school football days, the linemen had a drill. Lining up at one end of the eight-man blocking sled, we had to hit the first blocking pad, roll, quickly get in our stance, hit the next pad—until all 8 were hit. This was not too difficult except the other linemen would be hit-roll-hitting right behind you. If you were too slow, the others knocked you over. Those who got knocked over had to run laps.

Now, coach thought he was improving our speed and reactions. True. But he was also doing something else. He was teaching us *not*

to think. Thinking leads to holding back. In a game where an oppos-
ing lineman might be heavier and meaner, to hold back and think
means a missed or ineffective block and little or no yardage for the
ball carrier. It might also mean a trip to the hospital.

A stutterer doing street assignments has the same dynamic as
the lightweight offensive guard facing a big mean defensive tackle.
Stutterer thinks: 'This person looks grumpy, so I won't ask him.'
'This person looks in a hurry, so I won't ask him.' 'Aha! This person
looks nice, so I'll ask him.' Too much thinking. Too much holding
back. Too much avoiding. This leads to the classic Approach-
Avoidance conflict and FSDTA. Here's how to counteract the habit:

> *Our doubts are traitors, and make us lose the good*
> *we oft might win, by fearing to attempt.*
> WILLIAM SHAKESPEARE

To do the 15 Minute Sprint Drill, go to a busy street. Do your best to
make at least 40 contacts within 15 minutes. Forty new faces. Make
sure your questions can be answered quickly. The record is over
100. Keep at this drill until you get 40. If you can get 40 contacts
within 15 minutes, you can complete 100 within one or two hours.
No excuses.

Half Hour Costal Breathing Drill: This can be quite difficult for
those who are very busy, but some successful members of our
Programme will start the day just sitting up in a chair simply Costal
breathing. Some will also image the motion of the Diaphragm and
ribs moving as they breathe. The task, similar to meditation, is to
not let the mind wander. It is excellent for developing the ability to
concentrate. Try doing this for 5 minutes, then increase the time
until you can do a half hour or longer. But don't you dare think you
can forget taking a Costal Breath at least once every two minutes
throughout your waking hours just because you did your morning
Costal Breathing.

Reading Aloud: Many or most of us who stutter have tried to defeat
this monster by reading out loud. But it never worked because we
were practicing either outright FSDTA, or just being fluent. Now
you have the right weapons to win this war and get good playing

this sport. Reading out loud is very much like the tennis player hitting against the wall or ball machine, or the golfer hitting bucket after bucket at the driving range. So read aloud for at least 10 minutes a day until you reach that 100% confidence/0% fear. If you're really busy, it's probably better to do the reading out loud.

> *Practice does* NOT *make perfect.*
> *Practice makes permanent.*
> (USED BY MOST GOOD COACHES)

Talk to yourself: If you're alone, especially in your car driving, there's no law saying you can't talk to yourself, practicing all the techniques. This is especially good when preparing for a meeting, interview, confrontation, etc. and can help with Centering and Clarifying.

Use your cell phone: If you're around other people, either make a call to a practice partner, or pretend to call someone. Trying not to be too intrusive on the others, use this as an opportunity to show them you are someone working to overcome a stutter.

How long? Intensity & Persistence.

This process is much like taking an antibiotic when you have some kind of bacterial infection. You have to take the proper dose (intensity), and you have to take it long enough (persistence). If you take two antibiotic pills instead of the prescribed four per day, the bacteria will develop a resistance and the antibiotic won't work. If you stop taking the antibiotic for the prescribed time (because you feel better – see 'complacency'), the bacteria will develop a resistance and the antibiotic won't work.

If you do not use this method *intensely* enough, your stuttering will develop a resistance and this method will not work.

If you do not use this method *long* enough, your stuttering will develop a resistance and this approach will no longer work.

> *Perhaps the most valuable result of all education is the*
> *ability to make yourself do the thing you have to do, when*
> *it ought to be done, whether you like it or not.*
> THOMAS HENRY HUXLEY

Contacts: Quantity versus quality

There are times when you need to make many (like hundreds) of short quick contacts to overkill a feared word or sound. Once you have overkilled, however, there is still a need for contacts, but perhaps longer and not so many. Here are some guidelines:

Quantity (many and short contacts) –
Three things to consider:

1. When you have a sticky feared word or sound, you MUST take it to the boring stage. This is not negotiable. So far, the only thing that will do this adequately without drug or booze, is many phone and street contacts starting with the last word that gave you serious trouble. Start easy and work up to more difficult situations, but go for quantity and get each type of situation to the boring stage before moving on. Then go to the next feared word that gave you trouble, but you will probably find that it doesn't want to play anymore after watching you beat up its big buddy. Remember it is that first confrontation with a new face or new voice that will generally bring up the fear.

2. When street contacts are boring no matter what the situation or word, but you still have blocks in real situations. First you have to remind yourself of, and stand up for, your assertive rights of defeating stuttering in whatever real situations are giving you the trouble. Then you have to do phone and street contacts with whatever word gave you trouble in the situation. This is important, first to rebuild your confidence and second to see if your blocking has slipped from 'situational' to 'practice'. If you're still 'situational', then 10 quick contacts with the word(s) that gave you the trouble in the boring stage should do it for you. This would be 'putting in the wedge' if you were rolling a heavy stone uphill. If, however, you start blocking in 'practice', then you need to follow directions and get down to some heavy overkilling with many short contacts. Remember, if you are blocking in situations but not in practice, it is most likely an assertiveness problem where you have put the ring back in your nose and forgot that 'you have the right to do whatever is necessary to become a strong, eloquent speaker'.

3. Deliberate Dysfluency must be taken to the boring stage'. If you have any fear of Deliberate Dysfluency, then your foundation of 'assertive self-acceptance' is rotten and you will constantly be out of control.

Warning: Once your feared words and Deliberate Dysfluency are overkilled to the boring stage, *stop* making quantity contacts as this can now be counter-productive, using up precious 'juice' that may be needed when you hit more turbulence and need to overkill again.

Quality contacts: three things to consider

1. When you've overkilled all feared words to the Boring Stage, but have some discipline problems. Find contacts where you can speak longer, and really focus on technical stuff like long pauses, releasing residual air, good Deliberate Dysfluency, etc. Not just have an idle chit-chat using sloppy technique.
2. When you feel the need to push out your comfort zone. Again, you have already taken feared words and Deliberate Dysfluency to the boring stage.
3. **Testing.** Everything is great, but you want to see if some historical feared words want to come out and play. In military terms called 'search and destroy'. Make a few contacts using these old words that needed overkilling.

Combat fatigue

Combat soldiers – especially those who have lost battles or who are entrenched – need breaks. Otherwise they become fatigued and are ineffective as fighters. Occasionally, someone trying to overcome a stutter will have trouble with phone or street work or both. They continue to grab for tricks no matter hard they try, or how many situations they go into. Although there is some long-term benefit from simply attacking these situations, it can become counter-productive because tricks and avoidances are being reinforced.

If you are in this rut, drop down to an easier situation such as reading to yourself and practicing with friends and family. Do this constantly for a whole day. This means several hours while isolating and exaggerating everything on the checklist – especially the Big 4 (CB/HH/BR/DB). The next day, start out with a few 'hang-up drills' and hit the phone with much Deliberate Dysfluency. WARNING: Do not fall back on the 'combat fatigue' routine without a fight.

> *By perseverance the snail reached the ark.*
> CHARLES HADDON SPURGEON

Solidifying and polishing

You've overkilled feared words to the boring stage by doing 100+ contacts a day. Continuing to do 100 contacts, or even 50, a day will most likely become counter-productive as it will burn you out leaving no mojo for when you need to do some genuine overkilling. But, especially if you're fairly new at this and still need to bring it firmly to the 'Belief' stage, doing, say, 10 practice contacts a day including 'search and destroy' old feared words is a good policy.

A few times a month (again assuming you've killed your fear) it would be good to do 100 or more contacts, but more to solidify and polish your techniques and mentality. To help you do this, we have something from a former instructor (now a teacher) Heather Lucy:

Ratio Worksheet (by Heather Lucy)

Want to really know how you're doing? Take the time and effort to print out this worksheet to keep track of how well you do with each component. Some things to consider:

- **Decide, *before* starting your contact session, which items you are going to focus on.**
- **Fill in the top row of the Contact Ratio Worksheet with your chosen items** (or complete the already prepared one).
- **Decide, *before* doing an individual contact, which *specific item* you are going to focus on.**

- *After* each contact record your own evaluation by filling in the appropriate box with a + if you're satisfied or a – if not satisfied.
- **Look at your ratio of satisfied and not satisfied.** Is it better than your last contact session?
- **Make a note of feared words and keep challenging them!**

100 Contacts Ratio Worksheet   **Date:**

Item	FQCB	BR	HH	DBT	RTP	DD	AFS	RRA	EC	PT
1										
2										
3										
4										
5										
6										
7										
8										
9										
10										

Challenging words:	Number of + is
	Number of – is
	Ratio of + : – is

We've included 10 of the techniques/mentalities in the RW Sheet, but you can cross out and substitute others from the list below.

FQCB	Full Quiet Costal Breath
HH	Hit and Hold
BR	Block release
DBT	Deep breathy tone
RTP	Resist time pressure
AFS	Assertive first sound
EC/FP	Eye Contact/Focal Point
A	Articulate
PT	Perfect timing
F	Formulate
KMF	Keep moving forward
FR	Face Relaxed
HS	Head Still
SD	Shoulders Down

CHAPTER SEVEN:

Battle hardened – tournament tough

So you've drilled this new speaking technique until you are doing it in your sleep. And you've drilled your non-avoidance so much in the streets and on the phone that the police are looking for you. Now it's time to kill the monster. It is time to destroy his home.

A young recruit enters a Marine Corps boot camp. In this Rite of Passage, he is mentally and physically broken down and transformed from fun-loving teenager to warrior. He is issued a weapon and is trained how to use it. He participates in war games to practice using his weapon and tactics in battlefield conditions.

> *This is the true joy in life: the being used for a purpose recognised by yourself as a mighty one; the being thoroughly worn out before you are thrown on the scrap heap; the being a force of nature instead of a feverish selfish little clod of ailments and grievances complaining that the world will not devote itself to making you happy.*
> GEORGE BERNARD SHAW

He is not, however, a dependable soldier. He must now become battle-hardened. The only way to become battle-hardened is in combat. He must test his courage by facing death.

A General will battle-harden raw recruits by throwing them into a less important battle. Some military historians say that is why the untested American army first fought the superior German army in North Africa. The goal wasn't winning or losing, but to develop a core of combat veterans for more critical battles.

Tournament tough

It's one thing for a tennis player to hold on to his technique and game plan in a friendly match. It is quite another to do this in formal competition where winning or losing takes on a new dimension. Especially if you are on a team where your matches mean the difference between the team winning or losing. Muscles tighten. Thinking fogs. Here comes that easy lob. You hit the ball against the back fence. You'd never miss such a shot in a friendly match.

> *Winning can be defined*
> *as the science of being totally prepared.*
> GEORGE ALLEN

So formal competition is a different game. There is definitely a punishment for losing, and there is definitely a reward for winning. It is life's process wrapped up in a few hours. It is doubtful that immediate execution of the loser by firing squad would produce greater intensity. Even at the beginning level a certain amount of life and death is involved. The life or death of one's self-esteem. For a healthy person this 'death' is just a fleeting, half-second feeling. For an unhealthy person, the demoralization can last for days: it is much more than a stupid game.

A tennis player wants at least to play well in competition. To give his opponent a good match. To play well in formal competition a tennis player must become 'tournament tough.' How does one become tournament tough? PLAY A LOT OF TOURNAMENTS!

And just like the General throwing untested soldiers into unimportant battles in preparation for important ones, a tennis player will enter smaller tournaments in preparation for the bigger ones.

Someone trying to overcome a stutter also need to become battle-hardened, tournament-tough. Street and telephone drills are great for practicing your technique, assertiveness, and can reduce fear. They are like war games for soldiers and practice matches for tournament tennis players. But these are not the real battles. They are not real tournaments.

Real speaking battles are the core of your iceberg. Speaking tournaments have a consequence for your stuttering going out of control or reward for reasonable fluency. Dealing with people who you will never have to deal with again carries no substantial reward or punishment. What are real battle/tournament situations? Things like:

- In-laws (or prospective in-laws) are real battle/tournament situations.
- Potential love relationships are real battle/tournament situations.
- Job interviews are real battle/tournament situations. Speaking with your boss is a real battle/tournament situation. Speaking in class. Oral presentations at work.

These speaking situations are the 'big battles', the Grand Slam tournaments. You cannot stay in the trenches or clubhouse. You must prepare for these battles/tournaments and attack them. You cannot wait for these situations to come to you. You must seek them out. You do not wait for your boss to call you into his office – you call him for an appointment to speak with him (about anything). You do not wait for your mother-in-law to call you – you call her.

How do you prepare for major battles/tournaments? Answer: find a less stressful but similar individual situation. You must do some creative thinking, but here are some suggestions:

Arrange to speak with the mothers of some friends before contact with your mother-in-law.

Don't let life discourage you;
everyone who got where he is had to begin where he was.
RICHARD L. EVANS

Arrange some job interviews even though you have no intention of taking the position offered. Get accustomed to speaking to someone who has the power to hire and fire before you deal with the person who indeed has this power over you.

Practice speaking before groups by joining and attending speakers' clubs such as Toastmasters. This will help you become eloquent. You can find one through telephone information, the library, universities, etc. Locating one is good practice. If there is no speakers' club in your area, start one. It is a simple matter of placing an advertisement in local newspapers, sending letters out to companies, putting notices on bulletin boards. Toastmasters will send you guidelines for starting a chapter and running meetings.

Take a foreign language class. Although you will eventually be called to speak, you must volunteer to speak. Speaking in a foreign language is extremely good for your fluency as it requires more time during the pause (therefore more time-pressure resistance) to translate as well as formulate. Becoming fluent in a foreign language is part of becoming eloquent. It is fun, especially when you visit that foreign country.

> *Our greatest glory consists not in never falling,*
> *but in rising every time we fall.*
> CONFUCIUS AND RALPH WALDO EMERSON

Enroll in an acting class. Memorizing lines and putting yourself into a certain character can be very daunting, requiring immense focus and practice. You'll also have to polish your technique to sound more natural, and make sure any feared word or sound has been overkilled.

Warming up. Say you managed to get tickets to the Wimbledon Singles Finals and show up two hours early. As you are walking around looking in the shops to kill time before the match starts, what do you think the two players are doing? Watching cartoons in the players' lounge? No. They are on the back practice courts drilling forehands, backhands, volleys, overheads, serves, returns, etc. Then they spend some time just thinking and rehearsing their game plans. They might have a five-set match ahead of them, but they will still be out on the practice court for an hour. Why? Because it is important that every component of their game is 'tuned' before the points start counting.

> *Before everything else,*
> *getting ready is the secret of success.*
> HENRY FORD (1863–1947)

You, too, need to warm up before difficult speaking situations. This includes practicing the components of your checklist. It also includes knowing your subject matter (as much as possible) and how you are going to present it so that you don't get caught in the 'competence vs. incompetence' approach-avoidance conflict. It includes giving yourself some quiet time before the situation to center and clarify yourself using the 'Centering and Clarifying Flow Chart'.

Be in the process of Overkilling a feared word or sound. If you're battling a feared word or sound going into this tough situation, make sure you are at least making progress towards 100% confidence. You might only be in the barely manageable fear stage, but as long as you are improving through hard work and courage, you have a good chance of doing reasonably well. If you ignore the word/sound(s) and do not make any effort (or inadequate effort) to overkill, it will most likely tap you on the shoulder at the worst moment with a message that goes something like: *'Remember me? You couldn't say me yesterday even in practice, what makes you think you can say me now?'* So put some time and effort into as much overkilling as you can possibly do.

Regrouping. After the British were badly defeated in Western Europe, they evacuated their troops from Dunkirk and regrouped to fight again. After the Soviets were badly defeated during Hitler's Operation Barbarossa, they moved their weapons factories beyond the Urals and regrouped to fight again.

You might lose some battles in this war against the oppression of stuttering. You'll be in an important meeting or interview and will experience the freezing, struggle and distortion that will lead to another and another and another until you are grabbing uncontrollably for your old tricks and avoiding words. If you have been sailing on automatic for a while, it is probably too late to use Deliberate Dysfluency, image, focus, etc. This stuff must be practiced regularly if you want it to work in those surprise situations – but we all, except for those exceptionally disciplined, get lazy and overconfident.

The best thing to do in such a situation is be honest. Ask for a break, with (something like): 'Excuse me. I've been working to overcome a bad stutter, and it's coming back on me. Please give me a few minutes to get myself together.' Just acknowledging your role as a stutterer will take away much of the pressure – after all, your tricks and avoidances are just ways to hide this fact. Two circles start to overlap ... stress comes down.

If you can get a short break from the situation, do strong Costal Breathing with long pauses. Force yourself to image the Diaphragm in your Thorax. Remind yourself again to feel your voice coming deeply through your chest. Remember: the basic goal of this whole Programme is to get your speaking process down in your chest and articulate (even eloquent) speech becomes the by-product.

If your stuttering is still out of control after this, try to shut up. If you are stuck in the speaking situation, just do the best you can. As the German army in the Battle of the Bulge, your dying stuttering enemy has broken through your line of defense. You will need to acknowledge that THIS battle (not the war) has been lost. You must regroup, retrain, call in reinforcements and counterattack. Get your Ratio Worksheet, get on the telephone, go out in the streets, find another similar (but less important) situation and attack.

Good news and bad news. The good news is that, if you react immediately and intensely, your counterattacks will be successful and you will win the war. The bad news is that, if you do not regroup immediately and intensely, your counter-attack will fail and you will lose the battle (but not the war unless you give up).

> *What counts is not necessarily the size of the dog in the*
> *fight – it's the size of the fight in the dog.*
> DWIGHT D. EISENHOWER

CHAPTER EIGHT:

Crisis management.
What to do when things fall apart

So you've been flying high on automatic for weeks, months or even years. You thought the shame, guilt, self-hate and panic was dead and buried ... a thing of the past never to return. **Then it happens:**

Suddenly (probably a day when everything else is going wrong and your hexagon is screwed up mega in the negative) it hits you. You get *ambushed*. Perhaps it is something about the person behind the counter. Or something about the store's decorations. Or the colour of the hair of the person standing behind you. Who knows what will trigger it: Probably a combination of stimuli including your current state of mind.

> *Obstacles are things a person sees*
> *when he takes his eyes off his goal.*
> E. JOSEPH COSSMAN

Before you know it, those old feelings of terror well up from your subconscious. The old 'I'm not going to be able to get out this word.' You and your Diaphragm go into a giant approach-avoidance conflict and you have **a surprise return of the old Fear and an overwhelming reaction to Freeze, Struggle, Distort and/or use Tricks and Avoidances.**

But that's not the end of it. In spite of the warning that this would happen, the terror feelings are followed closely by feelings of discouragement and despair. Old tapes start again: 'Nothing I do will get the word out.' 'This method isn't working and will never work.' 'My stuttering is going out of control.' And so forth. **So what happened?**

Most likely (before the crisis) you had let yourself go back to speaking from the Crural Diaphragm while you were enjoying your automatic fluent speech. After all, non-stutterers always speak from the Crural Diaphragm. When the fear hit, your Crural Diaphragm went into its chronic contractions and it was too late to engage the Costal Diaphragm in the face of the surprise element, which led to panic. Then, although we have no scientific research to support this, maybe your lower brain couldn't decide between using the Costal or the Crural Diaphragm so it short-circuited the Phrenic nerve. (Or something like that.) Then that seemingly living nasty entity we call 'stuttering' brings up his reinforcements:

Despair and hopelessness

Think back to when you had tried everything to get words out. Remember the hopeless 'No matter what I do, I can't stop stuttering.' I personally remember the endless hours of reading out loud at night hoping that it would help me be fluent the next day – but it never worked even though I gave it my absolute best shot. Webster's defines despair as 'utter loss of hope.' Hopelessness. After so many experiences of these thoughts of hopelessness, it is small wonder that they remain even after we've reached that 100% confident stage.

There was a study done which verified that punishment-based learning is irreversible. And stuttering is most definitely punishment-based learning. You were punished (in some way) every time you stuttered. And the punishment strengthened the stuttering by strengthening the avoidance reaction. So it is possibly true that stuttering is not totally curable – but don't let this be an excuse not to work and fight.

So the feelings of 'nothing I do will help' will possibly be with you indefinitely. And these will come bursting forth like a visit from an unemployed relative with every FSDTA. The best thing to do is to realize that these feelings are just old tapes and TAKE ACTION.

Now, say you have experienced falling apart where you are once again mired in the swamp of tricks and avoidance. You had felt free but, like a bird in an oil slick, you are now having a very difficult time taking off again. You start your blast-off routine again. You put six hours and three hundred situations in one day. You go to bed improved, but still blocking badly. The tendency is to quit. Don't. Any athlete or musician who is facing a tough competition or performance after a long lay-off experiences the exact same thing. The first day usually feels terrible, but you just keep trying. The second day is usually much better, and gets increasingly better with every day of diligent practice. Trying to stop the FSD(TA) and feeling good about your speech after a bad fall will follow this pattern. The first day of practice will be discouraging. But if you push yourself and do your best, the second day should be much better. By the third or fourth day your high-point should be back – even stronger because you proved to yourself that you could indeed get your confidence back relatively quickly. Courage, as well as hard work, plays a big role here.

Rust, mess, fat, etc

Rust: Your car is being eaten away by rust. Big holes forming around the windows and under the doors. You take your rusty wheels to a body shop. The rust is sanded off, holes filled, anti-rust compound applied. Then the car is repainted and looks like new again.

Months later a spot of rust again appears. Not surprising as rust tends to have the same characteristics as cancer. If the spot of rust is not taken care of (sanded, anti-rust compound, new paint) it will quickly metastasize and your car will need another expensive trip to the body shop (or the junk yard) – which could have been prevented if you had taken care of the rust when it was a little spot.

The Mess: My ex-wife and I should have an award for being the world's messiest housekeepers. We both had sweet moms who cleaned our rooms because they wanted us to have time to do other productive things. So we never developed the habit of picking up after ourselves. Add to this two messy children and you have a certified disaster area. We had a cleaning lady who came in once a month. She kept asking for more money because our house was 'special.' After she'd worked all morning, the house was actually presentable. One hour later, however, it had returned to its original condition. Every so often I would attempt to reverse this pattern. It was like a religious experience. The neighbors knew it when they hear a certain scream coming from the McGuire house. I would go through the house throwing everything not in its proper place in a bag. Then I would dump everything in the big toy box muttering 'if they want it they'll have to dig around until they find it.' Then I give them the law:

'ALL FLAT SURFACES MUST BE EMPTY. ANYTHING FOUND OUT OF PLACE WILL BE DUMPED!'

It is amazing how good a house looks when there is nothing on the counters, tables, floors. Just a couple of crying kids who can't find their Barbies. 'A place for everything and everything in its place' my father always said. Then it happens: the half-eaten sandwich on the piano. The baseball glove on the table. The dirty socks on the couch. Like cancer cells, these quickly metastasize into an uncontrolled, overwhelming mess. In a few months the neighbors would again hear 'the scream' from the McGuire house.

Fat: I have a fat problem. It started back when I wanted to play college football. A 180-pound outside linebacker didn't have much of a chance in college. I needed to put on weight. Every night I went to the weight room. I also needed to eat more. Problem was, I was poor. Food costs money. So I got a job in the cafeteria. Every time the supervising cook wasn't looking, I stuffed my face. I remember the hard-boiled eggs. The chunks of pastrami and corn beef. The bread rolls. Everything and anything. Not that far removed from John Belushi in his famous cafeteria scene in the movie 'Animal House'.

So I quickly went from 180 to 210 pounds. But I couldn't lift weights fast enough (and study) to keep the fat off. Many fat cells were created. Although these shrunk when I later lost weight, they were always there waiting for the chance to fill up again. Every time my lifestyle changed to where I was not getting enough exercise, I got fat.

The pattern is always the same. The first extra pound. The second extra pound. The old 'I should go running now but I'm too tired.' The old 'I shouldn't eat this, but I deserve it because I've worked so hard – I need to replenish my energy ...' Soon, my size 34 pants and underwear are at the bottom of my closet, and I am shopping for size 36 – swearing that 36 is the absolute limit.

It would have been *so* much easier if I had taken care of those first few pounds immediately. Now I face dealing with at least 20 pounds of stubborn fat. Either another three month juice fast, or a slow painful diet both followed by a commitment to change my lifestyle including more exercise. At this point, however, I think I will go to my grave in my size 36 undies ... but my last words will have been at least articulate if not eloquent.

> *(Bad) habits gather by unseen degrees,*
> *as brooks make rivers, rivers run to seas.*
> JOHN DRYDEN (1631–1700)

You know what the comparison is: Take care of that first little spot of rust immediately and you don't have to take your car to the body shop. Take care of the half-eaten sandwich on the piano immediately and you can keep your house presentable. Take care of that first extra pound immediately and you don't have to go through another major diet.

So what is that first spot of rust? The answer is simple: it is a *word*. Of course! It is a stupid *word* which brings the fear, followed by panic, followed by the block followed (or preceded) perhaps by a trick or avoidance. And this word probably starts with a sound which in your dark stuttering past caused you the most trouble. More than likely it was a word which started with the first sound of your name.

TAKE CARE OF THAT FIRST WORD WHERE YOU BLOCKED, USED A TRICK AND/OR AVOIDED AND YOUR STUTTERING WON'T GO OUT OF CONTROL.

The return of your stuttering is not the result of some mysterious, incomprehensible demonic force. It follows the same laws as rusty cars, fat bodies, messy houses. *you* can maintain your fluency. Or *you* can go back to being a verbal cripple.

The battle of 'Dit'

I had been totally fluent for several months. Perhaps only a few little reminders, but nothing that threatened my precious fluency. Then it happened. I was trying to convince someone to buy one tennis string for his racquet rather than the other. In Dutch it was 'dit snaar is beter dan de andere.' Maybe it was because I wasn't being 100% honest (there was very little difference between the two strings.) Or maybe my time was up. Or maybe because I wasn't sure if the proper Dutch word was 'deze' or 'dit', which caused another approach-avoidance conflict. Whatever the cause, I seriously blocked on 'dit.' Much more than a 'little reminder.' When the customer left, I went to the phone and said 'dit is Dave McGuire ... etc.' After five blocks in a row, I saw visions of going back to slavery not to mention closing my Programme. The fear became intense, but I kept fighting. Finally it started coming deep out of my chest. I did about thirty extra phone calls each time beginning with 'dit' to make sure. Whenever the phone rang, I answered it with 'dit is Dave McGuire' rather than the usual 'Dave McGuire.' I went to bed relieved that I had gotten it back.

> *Diamonds are nothing more than chunks of coal*
> *that stuck to their jobs.*
> MALCOLM FORBES

The next morning however, I had another block on the same word. But I got it back down in my chest quicker this time and it stayed down for the rest of the day.

The third day, I had one or two mild blocks in the morning. I went into every stressful situation I could find using 'dit.' No blocks, no tricks. The three-day Battle of the Dit was over. I still felt fear when the phone rang, but the fear subsided after several times proving that I could indeed keep it down deep in the face of fear.

As with the Battle of the Bulge, it was a close call. **It started with a stupid three-letter word.** If I had not dealt with it effectively like I did, it would have spread to all 'd' words. Then to all hard sounds. Very soon, I would have had to close the Freedom's Road Programme. Because I won, others have won.

What can you learn from this? Several things:

1. Know the initial word that gave you trouble. In a feared situation, you might have blocked on several words, but it always starts with *one* word.
2. Respond immediately to this word. Do not procrastinate. If you go to bed that night without having given it your best effort, the problem will magnify the next day.
3. Keep pounding intensely at this word. It may take you days to kill the panic surrounding this word, but the fighting will keep it from metastasizing to other words. If you are half-hearted, the problem will increase. Be able to look yourself in the mirror every night and say 'I did my best. I fought my hardest.'
4. Do not quit. You may not make progress the first day. It might even take you a week of intense fighting. You will experience despair and discouragement, but don't let this be an excuse to stop fighting.
5. Dig up your 'Ratio Worksheets.' Use them.
6. If you get stuck several times on a feared word where you grab for tricks or avoid, drop down to less feared situations to practice. Then hit it again in the more feared situations. But don't stay in the trenches too long cleaning your weapon in an effort to postpone the attack while the enemy's tanks are rolling over you.
7. Go back and review 'Overkill' in Chapter 4.

The slippery slope
Going from out of control stuttering to strong, articulate, confident speech usually follows an exponential curve upward. Progress is slow at first then, if one works hard and follows directions, improvement is increasingly rapid.

Losing it also follows this exponential pattern. Regression is at first imperceptible, but (with increasing use of tricks and avoidance) quickly becomes a free-fall. If response is inadequate, you crash and burn. Then you have to start all over again.

Good news and bad news. The good news is that, if you take care of those first few feared words, you will quickly get your confidence back. Your speech will probably be stronger when you have proved to yourself that you can indeed get it back. The bad news is, if you don't take care of those words, the problem will metastasize and you will lose it again.

The forest fire

In 1985, I spent some time fighting a forest fire. Fighting a forest fire is about the closest thing to war one can experience. Like an infantryman in the rear trenches, I recall sitting in a fire truck half asleep watching battalions of soldiers – with their 'weapons' of shovels, axes, and chain saws – move up to the front line. Each fire-fighting company had its own uniforms with special emblems for the elite units of proven veterans. I could see the glow of the fire over the ridge and hear its faint roar. There was the roar, too, of water bombers. The driver, much experienced in this warfare, warned me that, should the wind shift, we could be fighting for our lives. In the meantime, our biggest job was staying awake.

The next day, groggy from 48 hours of no sleep, we went to the 'battlefield'. Fresh troops were still moving up to the fire line that had moved on. Our job was to 'mop up' the hot spots. Looking over the burned area, I could see small wisps of smoke rising from certain places. Occasionally, there would be a red glow or even a flame.

The experienced fighters showed me what to do. Dragging the heavy hose from the tanker truck, every suspected spot had to be dug up, doused with water, chopped up, doused again, turned, doused again. One would think that just a good turning and a little water would be sufficient. But it wasn't. There was still much burnable fuel on the ground plus dry areas that the original fire had missed. If these hot spots weren't completely extinguished another major fire could flare up again. Then a wind shift could set alight the unburned areas, trapping the fire fighters who were battling the main blaze.

Same with you after pulling out of a downward spin. You need to dig up every possible feared word or feared situation, douse it with every aspect of this method including Deliberate Dysfluency chop it up, douse it again.

Stall, Spin and Crash
So – regardless of the warnings – you let yourself get away with those first few tricks and avoidance. You are in a free-fall. You can barely speak a fluent word with your dog. The same thing happens to pilots. It is called a spin.

Back in my stuttering days I took flying lessons but quit because of one too many blocks on the radio. The approach-avoidance dynamics of my stuttering also tended to make me freeze during take-offs and landings. My instructor was getting nervous. But I learned something about pulling out of a spin.

An airplane has to keep a smooth flow of air over the wings in order to stay in the air. If (because of too steep a climb, turbulence, etc.) this airflow is disrupted, the airplane goes into a 'stall' followed quickly by a downward spin.

Student pilots are trained to put their airplanes into a stall purposely so they can practice pulling out of spin. The idea is to fly out of the spin. This means one must put nose down, put the throttle forward, and turn (still nose down) in the direction of the spin.

At first it is terrifying for the student pilot. If unsuccessful, he will die. But after a few successful pull-outs, however, the student realizes he can do it every time. Then pulling out from spins becomes fun.

But there's a catch: To successfully counteract a spin, a student pilot must respond quickly and intensely. There is not a whole lot of time to be slow and lazy.

And of course, pulling out from a spin is assuming the airplane has enough altitude. Which is why one must keep the throttle forward during takeoffs and why one must be very careful during landings.

So what are the parallels to stuttering? Should be obvious, but I will spell them out:

The Stall: If a pilot responds immediately to a stall, he will not go into a spin. If someone trying to overcome a stutter responds immediately to that first feared word, trick or avoidance, he will not crash into the swamp.

The Spin: Sometimes spins happen. If a pilot responds immediately and intensely (nose down, full throttle) to a spin, he will easily pull out if he has enough altitude and doesn't panic when he realizes he must go down before he can go up. If you respond immediately and intensely to severe turbulence, you will pull out if haven't fallen too low (altitude) and don't panic.

The Crash: The pilot will die if he can't pull out of his spin. You will not die if you can't pull out of your stuttering spin. You will just have to face the demoralization of having to start all over again.

On the following page is the 'Spin Pull-Out Checklist.' Use this as a guideline and evaluation of your response to a crash and burn..

Spin Pull-Out Checklist

In this war/sport, we all hit 'turbulence' where we lose confidence. If you do not react quickly and intensely enough, this leads to a fall where your stuttering will go out of control. The following is to help you evaluate your response to this relapse spin. Those who have not experienced such a fall should predict their response. Are you, have you been, or will you be:

1. Canceling every trick and avoidance?
2. Deliberate Dysfluency at least once per two breaths?
3. Using a belt to help with your rib expansion?
4. Taking at least two Costal breaths every minute during waking hours with pause, full inhale, full rib expansion?
5. Using the basic method with everything you say?
6. Dedicating at least two hours a day to practice (outside school and work) until you pull out of your spin and become stronger than you were before?
7. Increasing, if necessary, your practice time?
8. Getting up an hour earlier and going to bed an hour later, if necessary, to put in extra practice time?
9. Starting every morning with phone calls to practice partners if you have some?
10. Buying, reading, and utilizing all recommended books?
11. Taking responsibility for your difficulties (as opposed to finding excuses)?
12. Aggressively seeking out speaking situations?
13. Doing your best to resist the temptation to use tricks and avoid?

CHAPTER NINE:

How to lose it

Look at any stutterer who is still stuttering severely
or has relapsed and you see someone who has cheated
on the principle of avoidance reduction.
DR. J. SHEEHAN.

There are indeed laws governing stuttering, which are as unyielding as the laws of physics and chemistry. Unlike with social laws, the punishment for breaking these laws is fixed: you will continue to stutter uncontrollably, and you'll progress in the wrong direction towards the Swamp. There is no probation or suspended sentences. You will *always* have to pay the fine and/or go to jail. But what are these laws? Looking at the times that I and others trying to win this war started going down, here are 8:

The Laws

LAW NUMBER ONE: Do not use tricks.
You should know what tricks are by now. Old ones will keep trying to come back. New ones will try to develop. Be aware that tricks work wonderfully well when you've been 'clean' for a while. As with drugs and booze, however, tricks are a sure way to lose what you've gained. Don't fool yourself. You will never overcome stuttering and you will always go back to the swamp if you continue to use tricks.

> *The problem is not that there are problems.*
> *The problem is expecting otherwise, and thinking*
> *that having problems is a problem.*

THEODORE RUBIN

LAW NUMBER TWO: Do not avoid words or sounds.
Substituting a feared word or sound with a non-feared one will
elicit more fear and tricks. You will never gain 100% confidence,
0% fear if you continue to avoid words or sounds. Your fear will
always increase if you continue to avoid words or sounds.

> *We must travel in the direction of our fear.*
> JOHN BERRYMAN (1914–1972) 'A POINT OF AGE'

LAW NUMBER THREE: Do not avoid situations.
You may not be fluent when a television reporter sticks a micro-
phone in your face, but you must try. You might even use tricks in
such a tough situation, but it is better than running away.
Consciously avoiding a situation will increase your fear more than
anything.

If you do go into a tough situation and have many blocks, avoid
words and use tricks, make firm plans and preparations to go back
into this or a similar situation. This is like a tennis player who gets
beaten badly in a tournament increasing and intensifying his practice sessions, then signing up for and playing in another
tournament. He may get beaten again, but he repeats this process
until he rises to a higher level. He may never reach Wimbledon, but
he will at least reach his potential. He will at least be a competent
tennis player as you can be a competent speaker.

**LAW NUMBER FOUR: Immediately cancel violations of the
above laws.**
This is your 'fine.' The habits formed by punishment-based learning are very tenacious. And stuttering's tricks and avoidance are
most definitely the result of punishment-based learning – tricks
and avoidance are a response to fear. Therefore, even the

strongest ex-stutterer will experience those surprise situations, which will trigger the fear and will in turn elicit FSD and/or TA. Unless one is more than human, this will probably happen several times during your fight for speaking freedom. You can forgive yourself for it.

> *He that diggeth a pit shall fall into it.*
> OLD TESTAMENT: (ECCLESIASTES CH.10 V.8)

You cannot, however, forgive yourself for *not* canceling every trick or avoidance. And you must do it preferably on the same day it happens. The longer you wait, the tougher it will be. You can pay a small fine now, or wait and go to jail. If you do not cancel a trick or avoidance, this habit will be stronger and you will continue to use tricks and avoid and you will never reach the freedom of 100% confident, 0% fear, much less reaching Articulate Eloquence.

LAW NUMBER FIVE: Put in whatever effort is necessary.
You need to put out a certain amount of time and energy to improve. If you are not improving, then you must increase your efforts until you do. Once you've broken free of stuttering's gravitational pull (orbit zone) you can stay there with minimum effort. But until you break free, you must invest time and energy. You cannot be lazy.

> *There are no shortcuts to any place worth going.*
> ANON

If you are into a steep downward spin or have crashed, you need to put yourself back into WAR mentality, make this your number one priority, and use every possible waking minute to get it back. If you cannot get yourself going, and are a member of the McGuire Programme, you should return to an intensive course/refresher ASAP.

LAW NUMBER SIX: Respond immediately to turbulence.
Sometimes you will hit some situations which elicit a deal of fear. Especially if you deal with this fear with tricks and avoidance, you will quickly begin to relapse. The longer you wait to respond, the

farther you will have to climb back and continue your flight to freedom. Immediate response to turbulence must become a habit. If you continue to put off responding to turbulence, this procrastination will become a habit.

> *Fall seven times, stand up eight.*
> JAPANESE PROVERB

LAW NUMBER SEVEN: Respond intensely to turbulence.
If you respond to turbulence with an inadequate effort, you will continue to fall. The farther you fall, the farther you have to climb back. You must develop the habit of responding intensely to turbulence. If inadequate responses become a habit, low confidence and high fear will be your reward.

> *It is no use saying, 'We are doing our best'.*
> *You have got to succeed in doing what is necessary.*
> WINSTON CHURCHILL

LAW NUMBER EIGHT: Your response to turbulence must be long enough.
If you quit your intense response to turbulence too soon, you will fall back to your previous level of stuttering. Persevere.

> *'You can let yourself off the hook, but the laws governing*
> *stuttering will never let you off the hook.'*
> DR. J. SHEEHAN.

Mechanisms of failure

What do we need to obey the above laws? What do you need to go beyond stuttering to eloquence and hold on to it? Three things:

Work Ethic (including perseverance) to put in the work necessary to get good.

Courage to push out comfort zones, face feared situations and take reasonable risks. Courage to show people you are working on defeating your stutter.

Perseverance to keep working hard and being courageous for as long as it takes. Not just for a few days or weeks, but months or years or a lifetime.

You can fail to get what you want or lose it once you've got it with the same mechanisms with which anyone will manipulate himself or herself into not reaching or losing their goals. If we dive deeper into this, there are some other personality traits, 'mechanisms', or habitual behaviors or attitudes, that promote and maintain less than satisfactory work ethic, courage and perseverance. Here are five of the big ones:

Arrogance

You think you're too cool, intelligent, educated, rich, etc. to follow directions and work hard. Maybe you think you're smarter than your coach, know more about stuttering than the guy writing this book, make more money, drive a fancy car, live in a big house, younger, better looking, etc. Arrogance could be seen as the root of the following four traps.

> *When they discover the center of the universe, a lot of people will be disappointed to discover they are not it.*
> BERNARD BAILEY

Denial

Most everyone has heard of this before. Nothing new. An athlete will deny the fact that skipping practice or getting drunk the night before a game will negatively affect performance. An alcoholic about to come off the wagon will deny the fact that taking that one drink will put him right back in the gutter. A person trying to overcome stuttering will deny the fact that using tricks and avoiding words will cause more severe stuttering. Discounting or denying that the problem is really all that bad or that they are regressing. On another level, the whole game of stuttering revolves around denial and lying. I avoided words and situations and used tricks in an attempt to deny that I was a stutterer and to lie that I was a fluent speaker. It is small wonder that denial and lying carries over to other things, the biggest of which is denying that stuttering is indeed a *big* problem.

The alcoholic denies that a few drinks are really dangerous to his recovery from alcoholism. The stutterer denies that using tricks and avoiding (or not working to counteract FSD) will result in a quick trip back to the swamp.

Complacency

'This is good enough, I'm a lot better than I was before' is the message you give to yourself. You forgot that being good at anything means continuing to improve. Someone trying to lose weight will think 'well, I've lost 10 pounds. I deserve that googoo pie.' Of course, denial plays a role in this.

Intellectualization

You do your homework to find arguments against doing what needs to be done to get what you want. Arguing definitions and concepts. Challenging basic philosophies of the Programme and which rationale is valid instead of addressing the issue directly. Naturally you do this because you're smart, or think you're smart. (Arrogant?) Intellectualisers are constantly outsmarting themselves. If they put the same effort into just following directions rather than researching excuses to be lazy and not brave, they just might make some significant improvement.

> *Knowing is not enough; we must apply.*
> *Willing is not enough; we must do.*
> GOETHE

Commonly heard stuff from those who engage in too much intellectualization: 'What is addiction/trick-using really?' 'Is tightening up my mouth really a trick?' 'Is speaking fast really a trick?' 'This other (famous) Programme I was in uses syllabic/blended contact speech/etc., so it can't be a trick.' 'Overcoming stuttering is not really like sports.' 'It is simply not practical (fair and reasonable) to put this amount of time and effort into this.' 'Deliberate Dysfluency brings back my real blocks, therefore, this is not a valid technique, therefore I won't do it.' 'I heard so-and-so who is a coach has some big blocks. Therefore this approach is not valid (therefore I can alter it – incorporate tricks.)'

Externalization

The no-brainer stupid person's intellectualization. You simply blame someone else or something else for not getting what you want. Easy. Key word is 'responsibility'. .... not taking enough of it for your own mistakes and failures.

So okay. We all do these things at one point or another. It's when you do it too much so that too many things you want are not becoming realities that it's time to step back and take a look at yourself and what you're doing.

What to do about it? It's not rocket science. Just habits that need to be replaced with better, more productive habits. Build your character. Know these traps so that you can recognize them every time you feel yourself using these 'tools' to be lazy when you need to work, and being cowardly when you need to be brave.

Other things that keep us from winning this war

If the above are the tools that lead to not working as hard as we should, or not being as brave as we should, here are some personality traits that, if you have too much of these, can keep you from making the progress you want even if you are working hard and being brave. It is beyond the scope of this book to solve these for you, but there are many self-help books around as well as effective growth workshops and therapists.

Stress

We all know what stress is. Those who study it say it is caused by the classic 'flight or fight' response to danger. Sounds like an approach-avoidance conflict to me. Approach-avoidance conflicts in one part of your life will lead to the fear-of-stuttering approach-avoidance conflict. For the substance abuser, it becomes an excuse to start their drug use again. For someone trying to overcome a stutter, it becomes an excuse to start avoiding and using tricks again. Or to stop working.

A person trying to overcome stuttering is already under a great deal of stress. And stress has a direct connection to the Diaphragm. There isn't a lot of room for stress from other sources such as relationships, money, etc. Here are some aggravators of stress:

Perfectionism: Perhaps you see another stutterer who has attained fluency. You want to be totally fluent in every situation and you want it now. Not getting it now (or within your unrealistic deadline) or a surprise block triggers the 'I can't stand not being perfect' reaction and the old FSD and probably a trick and/or avoidance to keep up the façade (lie) of perfection.

Then you start looking for – and finding – excuses for why it's not working faster and more perfectly for you. This takes away from the concentration and effort required to reach eloquence. So your progress is even slower. You're in danger of throwing everything out the window and grab for your tricks and avoidance. Of course you'll have a 'good, valid' excuse for doing so.

A big part of perfectionism is wanting to be the star. The 'if I can't be on the first team, I quit (this is a crappy team anyway)' syndrome. Those who go faster than you probably have reduced their iceberg of feared situations more than you – probably because they did more non-avoidance training than you. Or maybe because they have spent more time developing their powers of concentration. And they are probably progressing faster than you because they are not dealing with the stress of perfectionism.

Low frustration tolerance: You fall apart under pressure. Any time you experience fear in a situation, you grab for tricks. You probably have great difficulty holding a focal point or Diaphragm image for any length of time. As with perfectionism, you are in danger of throwing the whole method out the window.

Excessive worrying: We all know about worrying. Sitting around thinking whether something you did was bad, or whether something you're about to do will be bad or good. Not taking action to resolve your doubts. Wasting time and mental energy that should be put into *doing* something.

> *If you want to test your memory, try to recall what you were worrying about one year ago today.*
> Rotarian

Resentments from the past

Probably applies more to stutterers than substance abusers. Stutterers have to endure tremendous disrespect. Disrespect leads to resentment. Resentment leads to stress. Stress makes unfreezing your Diaphragm more difficult, takes away from the energy you need to make progress with your speech, and takes away from your ability to concentrate.

What's more, this becomes a present-life pattern where some sign of disrespect will trigger disproportionate resentment. The old 'hashing it over and hashing it over' syndrome. 'What should I have said to that bastard?' 'What will I say when I see him again?'

You must first believe to the bottom of your heart that it is a destructive, stress-causing waste of time and mental energy. Go back and write down in detail every incident you can remember where you wallowed in resentment. Answer this: Did it help? Was it worth the stress? Was it worth the time? Did it ultimately hurt you?

Stuttering and substance abuse

If you are regularly depending on booze or drugs to get you through tough speaking situations, you are probably addicted or well on the road. This writer, in his stuttering days, has been known to take a few drinks before a difficult situation to be fluent. This writer's heart is irregular because he has also been known to abuse Benzedrine for the same reason.

If you have fallen into the abyss of substance addiction you need to deal with the addiction before attempting to deal with your stuttering. Get yourself into a good 12-step Programme. Don't wait until, like most drunks and junkies, you hit bottom. Or maybe you *need* to hit bottom.

Not addicted to booze and drugs, but perhaps overindulge? If you are trying to overcome a stutter, there are still dangers:

Danger number one When you are under the influence, you probably speak much too automatically, without a smooth Diaphragm movement. This is no problem unless there are situations which are causing blocks and trick using. It is especially dangerous if you are regressing.

Danger number two If you are struggling to reach a satisfactory level or fighting to reverse a regression, you cannot be nursing a hangover. There will be enough days when you are sick or tired from other things.

Top tournament tennis players, or any high level competitive athletes, go real easy on indulging, especially before a tough match. This Programme has seldom or never worked for people who are active substance abusers. Probably because whatever is causing them to abuse substances is compelling them to resort to the addictions of stuttering, namely tricks and avoidance. Advice? Get into a good twelve-step Programme and start controlling your substance addiction before tackling your stutter ... but, sometimes you can do both at the same time.

Desire for comfort and convenience
Unfortunately, conquering an addiction or stuttering requires one to come out of their comfort zone. Which is uncomfortable. Unfortunately, you as a stutterer are dealing with an affliction that is profoundly unreasonable and unfair. *You* need to declare total war on your stutter with special attention to the tricks and avoidance. War is never fair or reasonable.

Fear of doing something about a serious problem

Really committing oneself to treatment means having to admit that stuttering is a problem that requires a major effort to overcome. Some are afraid to face this. They are afraid that the treatment may not work. Or they are afraid it may work: Then they won't have an excuse not to realize their dreams and potential.

Minimizing the need for help

Someone whose stutter is once again out of control, who can't climb out of the swamp of avoidance mechanisms must admit that tricks, laziness, and avoidance are very powerful and he/she needs help from other people. Sometimes we just can't do everything ourselves.

Without a struggle, there can be no progress.
FREDERICK DOUGLASS

Friends (?)

Perhaps you are hanging around other stutterers who are not seriously working to eliminate their avoidance mechanisms. Perhaps they are not working at all. You underestimate their overt or, mostly, subliminal messages. Their messages will pop up in tough speaking situations when you need to practice but aren't feeling like it. Their verbal or non-verbal voices will be in the back of your mind. You will be more likely to lose your concentration, use tricks under pressure, or succumb to laziness when you need to work.

'One common slogan within Twelve Step groups is 'Stick with the Winners.' Many of those who go back to FSDTA do exactly the opposite. They seek out those whose ideas correspond to their own – and set up a 'support group for failure'.

Like a recovering alcoholic needs to get away from practicing alcoholics, someone working to overcome a stutter is well advised to stay away from those other stutterers who are practicing avoidance mechanisms. Perhaps when you have reach a strong level you can go help them but, until then, you need to save yourself.

> *A fool can always find a greater fool to admire him.*
> NICOLAS BOILEAU (1636–1711)
> *(L'Art poétique)*

Or perhaps you have a circle of fluent, so-called friends who have tolerated your company even though they have little or no respect for you: 'Tony the stutterer? Sure, he can come along as long as he doesn't try to say anything.' By struggling to keep these 'friends,' you are constantly putting yourself in the 'desire for acceptance versus fear of rejection' approach-avoidance conflict. If you are struggling for fluency, this conflict will lead to the fear-of-stuttering conflict.

> *Great spirits have always encountered*
> *violent opposition from mediocre minds.*
> ALBERT EINSTEIN

Face the music. They aren't your real friends. Dump them. Face the prospect of being alone for a while until you find new friends. Or maybe it will be one friend. Or no friends. No friends are better than the disrespect of being a tag-along. Nothing is worse than being dragged back into uncontrolled stuttering.

Or perhaps it is the controlling-type people who need the upper hand and therefore resent your becoming a fluent person. And they'll do things to undermine what you're trying to do. They will increase the time pressure. They'll say things like: 'I liked you better when you stuttered.' They'll not confront you when they see you use tricks. They'll help you find excuses not to practice and work. They'll help you avoid situations. They will continue to interrupt and talk over you.

> *No one can make you feel inferior without your consent.*
> ELEANOR ROOSEVELT

What to do? Take a class and/or read a book on assertiveness training. A controlling friend will either accept the new you on an equal basis or go their own way. Let it go. Don't try to hang on to it.

Aggressiveness

Once your speaking potential is set free, you will have a lot to make up for. Especially if you have had partial assertiveness training. The danger comes when you dump all those built-up resentments onto the wrong person like your wife or boss. Suddenly you are about to lose your job and getting nasty letters from your soon-to-be ex-wife's attorney. The stress caused by all this can lead to big blocks and, worse, an excuse to go back to your old ways.

> *How much more grievous are the consequences*
> *of anger than the causes of it.*
> MARCUS AURELIUS

Relationship change

It is very possible that your stuttering dictated your choice of relationships. These people very possibly need to control you and don't appreciate having to deal with a whole person now. They might very well put pressure (subtle or otherwise) on you to return to your controllable 'old self.' And the stress of the whole thing will offer you a great excuse to stop the fight.

> *Never be bullied into silence.*
> *Never allow yourself to be made a victim.*
> *Accept no one's definition of your life;*
> *define yourself.*
> HARVEY FIERSTEIN

Body changes

If you are successful with this method, you will experience a profound change in personality and probably a physical change. Many have experienced relief from chronic asthma, freedom from common lung infections, lowered blood pressure, more energy, etc.

But you can also experience perhaps heart palpitations from the excitement of a new life. Or you might forget to pause and hyperventilate. Or perhaps you'll forget to eat properly because of all the excitement of the new you.

Unwise decisions

Someone going through such a huge mental, emotional and physical change is in danger of 'going off the deep end'. You might be tempted to break up your marriage, quit your job, go on a buying/spending spree, take out a loan, etc. All this based on your (untested) 'new self.'

Don't. Stay cool. No big decisions. Wait until the dust settles. Your 'new self' is going to evolve constantly while you get used to being a normal speaker. This will take over a year. Big decisions based on you as someone who has been fluent for two months will probably not be the same as for someone who has been fluent for two years.

The danger is that the stress created by these chaotic decisions might very well become an excuse to stop working (if you need to continue to work), or to fail to respond properly when you are ambushed by the fear and panic.

Experimenting with tricks and avoidance

Tricks and various ways to avoid can be very sneaky. Maybe you'll clean up all your avoidance behavior, but you let yourself try something new and manage to convince (manipulate) yourself into believing that this new trick is not a trick but something okay to use. The new junk feels great and doesn't (at first) lead to falling back to using the old junk. Again, there's the old dynamic of the honeymoon period. Being clean of tricks and avoidance, like any addiction, for a while makes everything work better. The new trick worked great and didn't lead to uncontrollable stuttering. But the honeymoon, as it always does, ends and the dysfunctional relationship (with avoidance mechanisms) begins, followed closely by a return to uncontrolled stuttering.

Family problems

On the intensive courses and follow-up of the McGuire Programme, we emphasize the importance of family support and even participation. But sometimes, families can promote a return to uncontrolled stuttering and keep someone from getting back on track. Stuff commonly heard that undermines progress: 'Why do you have to speak in this strange way? You sounded so much better before you tried this method!'

Assuming you've tried to explain to your family what you are doing, they still disapprove of this new way you are speaking. They complain about having to wait for your pause, criticise your Deliberate Dysfluency, and make negative comments about the big Costal breath. Or, for married folks, someone who has worked very hard on their speech and experiences significant improvement becomes in many ways, a different person. Not the same person their spouse married. Unless the partner understands the process resulting from this (many times) sudden freedom, they could feel threatened. Some can perceive it as 'brainwashing' and take serious steps to undermine the progress.

We can only recommend (strongly) that you seek out a good marriage and/or family counselor and follow directions.

PART THREE

Stories from members of the programme

20 years on the programme

by Brendan Comport (United States)

(Brendan's first course was the original pilot group in 1994. He had his share of turbulence, but through hard work managed to become one of the most successful graduates. In 1996 he joined the United States Air Force attaining the rank of staff sergeant, got a degree in Engineering and is now working as a Civil Engineer in Seattle ... something he could have never done with his previous level of stuttering.)

I very distinctly remember the first course 20 years ago, and the first time I actually for once did not grab for a trick when confronted with a speech block. We were doing some practice drills in the class room around the second or third day and I had a major block. Up until that moment I was still in the do-anything-to-speak mode and quite effectively avoiding the words that I was afraid of. But Dave and the other students, thankfully, noticed my struggle and did not let me off the hook. I remember Dave said 'finally got you to stick with it!' I had been found out. No more being sneaky with my speech! Rather than grab for my go-to 'word substitution' trick, I gave the technique a chance and I battled to get the word out fluently. It all sort of hit me at once.

I remember a feeling of shock as I realized that, if I was ever going to be free of stuttering and the fear of speaking associated with it, I had to stop using that trick and all others. From then on there was never any doubt in my mind that the stuttering had to go. I began to see that it is all about overcoming the fear associated with stuttering. At first we need to work at becoming fluent even if our fear of speaking is high. Then with hard work and a generous helping of courage, we can push out our comfort zones and reduce that fear.

When I look back over the 20 years that have passed since first starting the McGuire Programme, it is apparent to me that the Programme has helped me with much more than my speech. It has certainly given me effective tools to have speech that is clean of stuttering and tricks, but in a larger sense it has helped me to develop a life that is largely free of the mediocrity and stress that came from using my stuttering as an excuse. Along the way I have met some fantastic people in the Programme, so thanks everyone way back then for not letting me off the hook! I hope I can do the same for other students.

The Danish bakery

by Andreas Ganderup (Denmark)

It's funny how I used to be terrified of the bakery in my town. Not necessarily because the baker was any grumpier than any other baker across the globe, but because I would be terrified of placing my order. My mom used to send me there every weekend to buy fresh bread for breakfast, and I never really got around to telling her how I felt about it because that would mean facing my fear and admitting openly that my stutter was a problem.

So, unaware of the psychological hell that she repeatedly put me through, she kept sending me to the baker. Every time I got there, I knew I wouldn't be able to order the Italian-style bread that she wanted because of my fear of revealing my stutter. Instead I kept buying another type of bread, and afterwards telling my mother that the others were sold out. As you can imagine, my mother was pretty annoyed at the bakery for always having her precious Italian-style bread out of stock no matter how early in the morning she sent me.

A few months after joining the McGuire Programme I revisited the same bakery. I felt the usual butterflies in my stomach but somehow I made them fly in formation. I was determined; there wasn't a snowball's chance in hell that I would let the same old stutter defeat me this time. I ordered exactly the Italian-style bread I wanted and I did it exactly the way I wanted to. That was a defining moment for me during my first time in the Programme and it has paved the way for many great accomplishments since then.

I still enjoy that Italian-styled bread from time to time – and luckily, they're no longer always sold out!

Tired of hiding

by Ken Bevers (United States)

As a covert stutterer, I often tried to hide my stuttering from the world. As a result, I always felt like I was making this huge sacrifice that few people knew about. I thought if I switched the words around here or didn't speak at this time, then I could preserve my pride and self-image. And I was right, but, shame, guilt, fear, loneliness, and helplessness became my true companions. The only reward I ever received from this approach was short-term comfort and safety. The trade-off was that moments of life and opportunities for success passed me by because I sat there feeling helpless.

The time I most vividly remember this feeling of helplessness was in college. My junior year of college I was the President of my fraternity and for a recruitment event had to introduce myself in front of a large group of interested freshman. I stood at the front of the room with the presidents from the other three fraternities, waiting to introduce myself. Of course, I had to go last. When my turn came I barely managed to scrape by with a ' . . . Annnnd I'm Ken'. No last name. No 'and I'm with Alpha Delta Gamma.' And though I was supposed to have said more I didn't. I was beyond embarrassed. At that moment I decided to do something about my stuttering.

Fast forward a few years of self-help seminars, fluency shaping, counseling, trying to not care, and many other approaches, and I still felt helpless. Then I heard about the McGuire Programme from watching a Gareth Gates video and decided to give it a try. Not long thereafter, I boarded a plane to D.C. where I was greeted by the lovely Maria McGrath and the suave Chris Cooksey.

At the end of that first course I felt so very different. The Programme gave me an opportunity to confront the fear I had felt for so long; the sports like approach challenged me to push out of my comfort zones and grab life and opportunity as it approached me; the support system resulted in new friendships and chances to coach other people; and the refresher courses built my confidence and strength over and over again.

Since that first course I have found much success in my endeavors. At toastmasters I have won awards and managed meetings. At work I have seen increased responsibilities and begun supervising. At home I have found enjoyment and comfort from knowing that I don't have to hide anymore. But, I have also met challenges. They say that nothing good comes easy and they are right. Yet I have overcome each challenge and, as a result, my view of the entire world has changed. What used to be hard lines of helplessness and permanency became malleable lines of hope and temporariness. My stuttering was no longer an inescapable set of chains, but a tool to move forward in life. And as my view changed I began to find passion and purpose in every day. Most importantly, I found myself becoming who I truly was all of those years.

This sea of change started the day I decided to step out onto what felt like nothing. And now I am able to go beyond stuttering ... to a place where I am living life on my own terms. I hope you take that step. Know that if you do, nothing will ever be the same.

Time for a change

by Scott Monson (Australia)

I joined the McGuire Programme in April 2007, having decided it was time to make a major change with my speech. As a manager, I was avoiding giving presentations and briefings to large groups. I would instead ask my staff to do it on the pretext of 'professional development', but really because I was too scared to do it myself. I realized that this was not the type of boss or person I wanted to be!

With a renewed hope that I could break free of the limitations of a life-long stutter, I embraced the need to not only use the tools and techniques taught on the intensive course, but to change the way I thought about stuttering. Following that first course I sought out challenging speaking situations to test my new skills and develop a belief that I could do many of the things I had avoided for most of my 35 years.

I joined a Toastmasters public speaking club, where I entered – and won – my first public speaking contest only seven months after joining the McGuire Programme. That was the first of many competitions I competed in – and won – at Club, Area and Division level over the following three years. I also approached service clubs, community organisation and schools offering to talk on stuttering, resilience and overcoming fears, and have given dozens of speeches in front of audiences of up to 300 people.

Now, seven years after my first McGuire Course, I am a professional executive coach, corporate trainer and public speaker – my voice is my 'tool of trade'. I spend my days speaking to people in a one-on-one or group environment, and have been invited to give key-note speeches at a number of national conventions. I could never believe that one day I would get paid to speak, and now it is how I earn my living!

I am also a Staff Trainer, Course Instructor and Primary Coach with the Programme, and have led courses in Australia, Mexico and New Zealand. The Programme has not only allowed me to exceed what I thought was ever possible with my speech, but to meet some fantastic people, develop treasured friendships and travel the world. What more could you ask for?

No longer ruled by the tyrant

by Russell Eden (England)

For over 25 years the words just kept getting stuck and every speaking challenge was a hugely fearful experience. In 2003 I reached a period of my life where I realized that something had to change, I could not go on any longer being ruled by my 'demon stammer'.

I attended my first McGuire Course in August 2003 and discovered a level of freedom to speak, beyond my wildest dreams. I have never looked back; my speech control and overall confidence in all speaking situations continues to develop and grow.

I now have a job that I really enjoy; helping people with varying disabilities that are unemployed, find a route in to sustainable employment. The job is primarily a training role and every day is a really exciting and rewarding speech encounter.

I never thought I would be able to speak in an articulate and eloquent manner with such a fantastic level of control over my stammer. And today ... this is now a reality.

Life is really exciting and speaking no longer commands an overwhelming fear. Anything is possible if you work hard, believe in yourself and never give up on your dream.

The best medicine

by Alan Badmington (Wales)

I was in intense pain; my back had been causing problems for several days and I could not sleep. We had just returned home from holiday, where the non-supportive bed had been unsympathetic to my medical condition and I was still suffering the consequences.

Wearily, I made my way to the doctors' surgery; I required something to alleviate the extreme discomfort. The usual pills had failed to have the desired effect and I was in desperate need of relief. As I sat in the waiting room, it was rather ironic that I dozed intermittently. My eyelids seemed as though they were implanted with lead; I felt absolutely drained and devoid of any energy.

My usual GP was unavailable, and so I had no alternative but to accept the first appointment offered. The doctor, a youthful female locum, appeared quite attentive as I explained my predicament. But, for some reason, I felt uncomfortable. Could my poor physical condition be affecting my speech?

The supreme confidence I had exuded since joining the McGuire Programme (just three months earlier) had, momentarily, evaporated and I sensed that certain tricks (which had been such a trait of my life-long stutter) were attempting to return. It was extremely disconcerting; I could not understand what was happening.

I succeeded in explaining the circumstances of my medical problem without too much difficulty, although I was convinced that I may have practised minor word substitution. I had promised myself that avoidance was a thing of the past and now I was succumbing

to temptation. The medical practitioner duly handed me the pre-
scription I had sought and I bade farewell. I felt crest-fallen and
insecure as I left the surgery; my self-esteem and confidence tinged
with fragility and doubt.

Upon my return home, I reflected on the occurrence; deeply
concerned at my performance. Had the bubble burst? Was this the
start of a regressive journey down the slippery slope? Fortunately,
I was not permitted to dwell on the matter any further, as I sought
the refuge and comfort of my own unyielding mattress. Within seconds I was asleep.

When I eventually surfaced, the painkillers had performed their
purpose and I felt surprisingly refreshed. Despite the obvious physical improvement, the memory of the unpleasant surgery
experience was still uppermost in my mind.

I knew that I could not move forward until I had eradicated the
setback I had experienced. In McGuire terminology, it was essen-
tial that I practiced cancellation. Within minutes, I made a
disciplined telephone call to the surgery to arrange another
appointment for the following day. Not only that, I insisted on
being allocated the same doctor, at a time identical to the original
encounter. If I was going to cancel, then I wanted to do it with
style. I needed to re-create a similar set of circumstances (albeit 24
hours later).

At the appointed hour (9.30am), I entered the same surgery,
where I was greeted by (yes, you've guessed) the same receptionist.
I occupied the same seat and waited for the same GP to call my
name. She appeared surprised, as I deposited myself in the chair
before her, and enquired if there had been any improvement in my
back condition.

Resisting time pressure, I paused, secured eye contact and
acquainted her with the fact that I was trying to overcome stutter.
Outlining the purpose of my revisit, I apologised for taking up her
valuable time, but stressed the importance of cancellation.

I believed that my wellbeing was at stake and felt totally justified
in enlisting her aid to resolve what I considered to be a genuine
health problem. Would she view it in the same light? I fully
expected some kind of admonishment (or, at least, a display of dis-
pleasure) but, to my amazement, she exhibited considerable
interest and developed the discussion further. We spoke for at least

25 minutes, while I related my experiences of the McGuire Programme, and acquainted her with some of the contents of the course manual, 'Freedoms Road'.

Indeed, when I suggested that I might incur the wrath of her backlog of waiting patients, she made it clear that she would much prefer to continue with our oral exchanges, rather than fulfil her mundane consultations. As we parted, the accommodating medical practitioner confided that I had 'made her day' and requested literature about the Programme. 'Don't hesitate to come back at any time, I'd be delighted to see you', she added.

I thanked her profusely for her courtesy, patience and understanding, but diplomatically stressed that I hoped my future visits would be few and far between. We laughed, shook hands and I left the surgery feeling ten feet tall. (Indeed, I had grown in stature to such an extent, that I have a distinct recollection of bowing my head slightly in order to negotiate the consulting room door).

That visit proved invaluable; the original episode had caused me a great deal of consternation, and it was imperative that I replaced it with a positive occurrence. Had I not orchestrated a cancellation, then I have no doubt that the former uncertainty and fear (which preceded my McGuire days) would have festered and multiplied.

Stuttering is an interactive, self-perpetuating system of components, which thrives on bad experiences. It is fuelled by the memories of unpleasant speaking difficulties (and associated situations) that have accumulated throughout our lives.

After joining the Programme, (and, finally, experiencing the removal of the inhibitive oral shackles), I vowed that I would never again nourish and sustain the debilitating demon that had so adversely controlled my life since childhood. I knew I had to arrange an action replay, without delay, in order to redress the balance, and get back on track.

The 'Laws of Stuttering' had been contravened on two counts (using tricks and avoidance) and implementation of Law 4 (cancellation) was the best (and only) medicine. The outcome was just what the doctor ordered, allowing me to continue my successful passage to 'Articulate Eloquence'.

Another story from the first group

by Ron Evans (United States)

Hello. I'm Ron Evans, a participant in the April 1994 'Self-Help Stuttering Programme' held in Dave's home town of Santa Barbara, California.

Let me start by saying, 'Thank you', first and foremost to Dave, and second to Dr. Ronald Kapp, who made the course legally possible by coupling it with his medical research. Over the past 20 years, that single course has had a tremendous positive impact on the quality of my personal and professional life.

I don't remember how I found out about the Programme, but it seemed promising and didn't require a lot of time, so I made the 90 mile drive from Long Beach to Santa Barbara, not having any idea what I'd find there. What I found was something astonishing and miraculous – a method that turned stutterers into fluent speakers in less than one week.

The participants' severity varied greatly, from some who contorted their faces trying to force the words out, to others who only stuttered under certain conditions. I was in the latter group, stuttering primarily when doing things like ordering over the phone, introducing people, asking clerks if they had a particular item, ordering food, and making presentations. I had been stuttering a long time, and had gotten proficient at substituting words in mid-sentence. Later, when I told people about the course, they often replied 'I didn't know you stuttered', but I did – sometimes a lot.

Dave knew the way to 'beat the monster' (as Dave put it) was the same for all of us regardless of our severity; we all went through the same set of drills with no slacking off. Dave passionately applied athletic coaching techniques to motivate and challenge us to quickly learn and apply his method. One of the highlights was wading chest deep into the Pacific Ocean to prove we could still keep focus and cycle through the steps correctly, while shivering and watching out for the next wave. That showed us we were capable of staying 'in method' no matter what was going on around us.

By far, the hardest thing for me was phoning a total stranger and stuttering on purpose. I had spent years trying to avoid the embarrassment of stuttering, and now Dave is telling me I need to stutter to another person. I feared it, and absolutely did not want to do it. But I did. I called a local auto parts store and asked if they had a certain part in stock, stuttering for probably 3 minutes to answer the man's simple questions about the make, model, year, engine, etc. He was very patient with me, and at the end when I told him it was an exercise for a stuttering class, he was supportive and encouraging. Here I had just wasted part of his work time, and yet he was kind and supportive. Amazing! Gee, maybe most people are like him, and there is really nothing to fear. Maybe I hadn't been giving people enough credit.

In the years following the course, I have stuttered on occasion, but have always been able to 'counterattack the monster'. It is a great feeling.

Alcoholism and stuttering

by Charlie Caselton(UK)

I'm an alcoholic – no, I'm a drunk. I prefer to say 'a drunk' because it keeps me more in touch with where I was. Although alcoholism is a clinical condition 'alcoholic' sounds way too mature and respectable for a young man like myself, so let's just stick to 'drunk'. Before I stopped drinking the thought of going a day without alcohol was impossible, unreasonable, inconceivable and downright unnatural – yet here I am, I haven't had a drink for five years and that feels great. Throughout my recovery from alcoholism I've found the tenets of AA to be closely linked with, and highly applicable to, how I view my ongoing battle to overcome stuttering.

Alcohol always held a particular attraction for me I had learnt from my early teens that alcohol gave me extra confidence and loosened the tongue – what more could any stutterer want? It was the perfect substance: relaxing, intoxicating and FUN. While I consider my stutter as being a contributing factor in my drinking, it wasn't the only reason, but if you're an alcoholic – who needs reasons? I could drink on any excuse, in fact there were no excuses I didn't drink on. However I believe that, stutter or no stutter, I would have become an alcoholic anyway – I'm just grateful I was forced to realize it at 29 rather than 59.

Alcohol wasn't always a problem. It was only my last three years of drinking when I really felt imprisoned, but my stutter has always been a problem to me. It feels like I've forever been a captive held under mouth arrest. From the very first days stuttering robbed me of my dignity. Alcohol, if you're a practising alcoholic, also robs you of your dignity, but before it does it will have been a friend; a false friend no doubt, but a friend nevertheless – comforting, soothing, strengthening. My stutter was never a friend. In past speech therapy groups I have been asked to name the benefits of stuttering. I could never find any. One possible benefit mentioned by others has been that stutterers use their stutter to stick out from the crowd. This argument always struck me as laughable and rather offensive. There are many other ways of sticking out from the crowd; academic – or any sort of – excellence, sporting prowess, achievement, hell, even fashion sense or some wacky haircut. Perhaps there are stutterers who use their stutter to help them stick out from the crowd, but I suggest that if they are that limp of brain and attitude, and they are using their stutter for this purpose, then perhaps they deserve to stutter.

During my first few months in sobriety I often thought about my stutter and why, if I, a drunk, could stop drinking why I, a stutterer, couldn't stop stuttering? After all they are both learned behaviors and as such can be unlearned. They are both things that you do, rather than things that are done to you. Some stutterers may disagree with this last statement but I strongly believe it is true. In both conditions it is easy, and is perhaps part of the initial process, to see yourself as a victim, to throw up your hands in horror and despair and wail 'Why me?' The question 'why me?' is really irrelevant. What is relevant is the belief that we can change. That is the wonderful thing about human beings – our capacity for change, our capacity to improve. As I said at the start, before I stopped drinking I would have thought it way beyond my capability for a day to go by without my taking a drink. It was a concept that was out of this alcoholic's then tenuous grasp on reality. I used to think the same thing about stuttering.

Stutterers use many tricks to appear fluent and to maintain fluency once started. They avoid (or substitute) words, sounds and situations, often preferring not to speak altogether to preserve the image of fluency. They speak too fast, they speak too slow, or they begin speaking when the other person hasn't finished. They tap their feet, click their fingers, nod their heads, close their eyes, yawn. They speak too softly, too loudly or without emotion. The variety of tricks used is akin to the variety of drinks drunk. There are literally thousands of them. They can be shaken and stirred into all sorts of cocktails so one might try, say, avoiding a word AND speaking too fast or tapping your feet and nodding your head. Using tricks is a bad and dangerous habit and as with other dangerous habits the tail often ends up wagging the dog. What starts out as a seemingly harmless habit to help you out of trouble becomes an addiction destined to create trouble. On the first morning of Dave McGuire's course four of us were having breakfast at the hotel. There were two Germans who rabbited away fluently for 15 minutes without a break. Not a single stutter or hesitation did I hear. I marveled at, and envied, their fluency and seriously wondered if I was on the right course – these people were fluent, what could they be doing here? Sitting with the two seemingly fluent Germans was a silent Scotsman. I sat at the other end of the table. I later learned the two Germans were masters of avoidance. These two could have avoided for Germany on the international stage without fear of embarrassment. They maintained their fluency by adeptly avoiding/ substituting/ changing all words they might have trouble with. Even though they appeared fluent and eloquent they were just as enchained as more visible stutterers. The Scotsman and I both maintained our fluency by not speaking. There is something dreadfully ironic about that isn't there? – maintaining fluency by *avoiding* speaking.

Avoiding and using tricks is something we would rather not do but nevertheless feel compelled to do. As a practising alcoholic I would wake up every day swearing that today I would not drink, yet a few hours later I would find myself propping up the bar with a pint of Guinness in my hand. Admittedly I would often feel slightly bemused as to how I got to the bar and came to be standing there with a drink in my hand when I had sworn off drink, but that goes to show the power of addiction. How often have stutterers sworn off avoiding/using tricks yet still find themselves, mid-block, wondering how they came to be there? I chose, against my will and my best intentions, to have a drink in the same way that I choose to avoid/use a trick. Even though that part about choosing to use a trick (no matter how involuntary it appeared at the time) always made sense to me, it was difficult to accept. I have found that accepting that fact was crucial in the way I feel about my speech. If you can choose to avoid/use a trick then you can choose not to. You can also choose to stutter. Many people, myself included, have found Deliberate Dysfluency to be very helpful. Deliberate Dysfluency, which I don't do enough of, takes the fear out of speaking because instead of hiding the stutter (the intention of the majority of stutterers) you accentuate it. Deliberate Dysfluency puts you back in the driving seat. It works on the principle that by intentionally doing something that you fear, the fear will decrease dramatically. To a stutterer who has never heard of Deliberate Dysfluency, this technique may appear out of the question. **'What? Show my stutter . . .? On purpose? – No. No no no no no no no'**. I've found Deliberate Dysfluency a very effective tool in reducing tension and, somewhat perversely, becoming more desensitized to my stutter.

A major difference between overcoming stuttering and my recovery from alcoholism is that recovering from alcohol is a lot more clear-cut. In AA one is constantly reminded that alcohol is cunning, baffling and powerful. But it is nothing compared to the use of tricks which are all of the above plus sneaky and seductive. You know if you pick up that first drink that you've started drinking again. End of story. Whereas with tricks, oftentimes I wouldn't be aware that I had used one until someone pointed it out to me, or until I started to tape and playback my conversations. So sometimes one isn't even *aware* of the tricks creeping in until afterwards. If a recovering alcoholic picks up a drink he/she will know they've done it. They might be surprised to see the drink in their hand, but they'll know they put it there. They won't have to wait until afterwards to plead ignorance. The one time I've even come remotely near picking up a drink was by mistake. Instead of picking up my glass of ginger ale I picked up my friend's beer. As I tipped the glass back to take a drink my nostrils were assaulted by this vile smell and I quickly put the glass down before I could take a sip. That was a reflex action, an action I am building into my speech pattern to alert myself to the danger of tricks as my nostrils alerted me to the whereabouts of alcohol. Take it from me, once you stop drinking, beer goes from being the amber nectar to resembling nothing more than stale piss.

Alcohol was an easier enemy to fight because its effect was so apparent. I knew that alcohol was making my life totally unmanageable, I knew that I couldn't carry on drinking, so I knew what had to be done. I might have drunk because I had problems but I had more problems because I drank. With my stutter, yes it has certainly added a painful, immensely frustrating element to my life and, yes, I've often felt my life has been stifled, restricted and impeded but we learn to live with it, we learn to cope, we *have* to cope. In that sense our lives weren't unmanageable, often unbearable perhaps but we could fashion some sort of (dis)order out of our existence. That's the self-image that we've created. Because we rarely see or hear ourselves our views of ourselves can be softened. It is only on the rare occasions when we see ourselves on video or hear ourselves on tape or spy ourselves in the mirror, midblock, on the telephone that we realize the extent of the discomfort we must put our listener under. It is then we really see the unmanageability of our lives. We can't manage our voices, we can't manage verbal communication or expression, we can't pretend things are OK and that our stutter doesn't really affect us. That is when the effect of the stutter reappears and we, oftentimes, resolve to get back into speech therapy.

My aim is to duplicate my aversion and strong feelings about my using alcohol onto my using tricks. I was fortunate in that the obsession to drink left me fairly quickly. Not drinking has been relatively easy. It is not something I seriously think about because I know that for me, alcohol isn't an option. It just isn't an option. I know that to drink again would be a huge step backwards, a step towards some truly horrible feelings. A step to immediate pain, anger and despair. I'd do anything to avoid those feelings and not pick up that first drink. I'd rather be tied naked to a post in a frozen midwinter field and pelted with rotten tomatoes than pick up a drink. If I did drink again the guilt would be overwhelming and that makes it easier not to pick up that first drink. Also the thought of going back into a clinic is aversion therapy in itself.

There are many aspects of AA philosophy and AA sayings that I find I can usefully apply to my battle with stuttering. Having substituted trick for drink, one saying becomes: **'One trick is too many, a million isn't enough.'** A basic part of AA life, particularly if you've just stopped drinking, is the requirement to go to meetings. Going to meetings serves many purposes. It stops you drinking for that hour and a half. It keeps you in the company of other recovering alcoholics who, nearly always, have the answers to your questions. It gives you hope because you see how many other, formerly hopeless, alcoholics don't have to drink. One of the great things about AA is the number of meetings available to recovering alcoholics at all times of day wherever you are in the world. While there are, as yet, not enough of Dave's former students to be able to have daily meetings, I regard staying in daily contact with them and Dave, and doing speech practice on the phone as my version of meetings. An AA saying I've heard many times is, 'When you least feel like going to a meeting, that is when you should go'; i.e., when you're finding all sorts of excuses (lazy, tired etc.) not to go to a meeting that is when you should make sure that you go. I feel the same way about my phone/speech practice. When I least feel like getting on the phone, when my excuses crowd in and try to persuade me that there are really many other things I should be doing (like watching TV) THAT is when phone practice/contact with former students is really going to pay off.

Another factor I was told about in AA that really helped is that you have to be selfish about your recovery. You have to put what you need to do above anyone else's. Look after #1. Stick with the winners and don't associate with those alcoholics who are still drinking. It'll only lead to more pain and who needs that? That was an easy thing for me to accept because I was adamant that nothing and no-one would negatively affect my recovery from alcoholism. If you stick with the winners some of their magic might rub off on you.

The belief uniting stutterers and alcoholics is the sneaking conviction that their condition keeps them in a place where they know they don't belong. 'If only I wasn't an alcoholic I would . . .,' and it's true if only you weren't an alcoholic you would! Since I've stopped drinking I've done things I would never have believed myself capable of doing if I'd been drinking. In my battle against stuttering I'm already doing things I would never have attempted before going on Dave's course. Of course I've set myself much higher goals but I see overcoming stuttering as an ongoing thing. I know I'll get there. I know I'll achieve all my goals. Hey! I have a dream as well – one day we will all be free. *'Free at last, free at last, hallelujah! Free at last!'*

The entrepreneur

By Bill Windsor (Australia),

First course: February 2000. I am a graduate from the March course in Brisbane Australia. I have fought my stuttering for 40 of my 53 years. Like many fellow stutterers, I gave up on formal education and great opportunities presented to me because of my speech.

At thirteen I began to treat myself. At this stage I could not put two syllables together. On the advice of an old radio announcer I began reading to myself in the mirror, using a metronome speaking in a timed rhythmical manner.

When I blocked I would see that my mouth, tongue, lips were in the wrong shape so I would stop and start again. By the time I was 16 I had obtained reasonable fluency and I was overcoming the fear of social situations although I never used a telephone until I was 21. About age 17 I involved myself with a group therapy Programme run by the Queensland education department. This group was run by a team of young therapists who used the methods of the day plus involving us in real social situations, going to restaurants, shopping and the like but never actually dealing with the fear and anxiety that we all experienced, particularly as young adults. However I found a type of use Deliberate Dysfluency they taught very useful so I added it to my growing bag of anti-stutter tools, but for me it was back to my reading and mirror treatment.

At 19 I began my own business because I was too afraid to apply for a job and employed a secretary to do the phone work. I was 21 before I used a phone. I could tell stutter stories for hours at this point but at this point I must say that I was overcoming the fear of social and business situations, but I knew there was something mechanical in my speech that I was not getting a handle on and that happened by accident 20 years later. In late 1999 while in Memphis Tennessee I had a chance meeting with Page Farnsworth a speech therapist who introduced me to the Stuttering Foundation of America. I began to talk to Page about the fear that stutterers have of the simple act of speaking and how if you have never had the problem you can't begin to know what it is like. I began to read every bit of information that she gave me. At that very time I received videos sent to me by my friends at home of the course in my home town of Brisbane.

In the late 80s I met a wonderful soprano who changed my life in many ways who pointed out to me that I did not breathe properly and fully particularly when I spoke, so when I saw the videos on the McGuire Programme I immediately flew home and annoyed the hell out of Rita Savva until she could fit me into a course. I was enthusiastic about the course because it was run by stutterers developed by stutterers and not by learned clinicians. In my daily life I have always listened and taken advice from those who have achieved in their field of endeavour and not taken so much advice from the so-called expert professional. I had no idea what the Programme entailed, but I knew that I had to learn to breathe.

Somehow it was all starting to come together. I also had no idea that it would be so physically demanding. Having played a lot of sport and being involved in business I appreciated the need for the discipline, which the Programme calls for. It is not easy but the results are fantastic. The cloistered environment of the course shows us what we and others with our differing degrees of stuttering can achieve with total commitment. I began the last day of my first course crying uncontrollably at 5 in the morning, thinking of my dear father and how his life would have been so much different if he would have had the opportunity that we all had. He stuttered very badly till the day he died. It was also tears of joy for a young lad Adam from Kyogle just near my dad's hometown of Coraki who now had the rest of his life to overcome his stutter and so make a total commitment to his own future not held back by the fear of speaking.

My first course has taught me more than how to defeat my stutter. Resisting time pressure has taught me to listen better, relax more during stressful times and give more considered opinion to what I am about to say. The support group that has followed the course has shown me that I am not the only one that battles with the difficult days. For me, the follow-up and daily contact with my coach has proved invaluable. The sharing of our daily speech problems helps us all. I speak quite a bit to groups and even though it is only a month since my first course people who have known me for a long time can notice a difference in the way I am speaking. For me, I no longer fear the introductions. I will not have to change my wife's name from Carolyne to Ophelia or move the two houses from Wynnum to Manly, if I really want it I have the combination to defeat the stutter. Since the course my speech has had its good and bad days but I remember when learning to box they taught us all the individual aspects and how difficult it was to put that combination together while at the same time avoiding being hit by your opponent. This technique is so much the same, putting the combination together. I'll just keep working on it and doing my best. Traveling as much as I do both in the USA and at home I have met many people with our shared disability from all walks of life some like myself believe we have succeeded because of our stutter, it took us out of our comfort zone, while others have withdrawn from the speaking world, but the one thing we all agree on is that we would rather not have it, or the fear of it being in control of our speaking situation. The McGuire Programme gives us the tools and structure to be totally in control of our stutter, to defeat it both in the long and short term.

Offloading baggage

by Michael Hay (UK)

I'd like to share a story with you about my biggest speaking situation yet which happened this morning. I gave a speech to 600 people at my old school assembly.

Now, although I have done Live TV interviews before this was my biggest situation because it was also my biggest cancellation. There was an incredible amount of emotional baggage attached to it. When I was seventeen, I was a prefect in my school and one of the duties is to give a reading at the morning assembly in front of the whole school. I avoided this completely as it had petrified me and it has been gnawing away at me ever since for the last 8 years. When I started the McGuire Programme I knew you were recommended to cancel things and I recognized two main situations that I had avoided which I could go back to cancel: 1) a bible reading at my Church which I had been asked to do, and 2) this reading at my old school assembly. I cancelled the Church one quite quickly, but for two years now I have been avoiding canceling the school one. I have made every excuse under the sun as to why I wasn't able to do it.

In Newcastle this September, in the split session on the Sunday morning, Terry Cardwell asked everyone to stand up and give themselves a goal for the coming week. Some said they would use the phone list more, but something told me to use this opportunity for something bigger. I stood up and said I would cancel out my biggest avoidance from my past – my school reading. I don't know if I would have managed this on my own. It shows how powerful the support and motivation from others around you can be. That atmosphere gave me the guts to stand up and make that promise. After I had made that promise in front of everyone there was no going back. No question. No excuses.

I did the reading this morning. It went very well. I got an email from the headmaster later this morning, which said 'I thought the content and delivery of your speech was magnificent'. I have let other McGuire grads hear the speech on my Dictaphone and they have said it was great. Although I am on Cloud number 9 right now, however, I wasn't as excited when I came off the stage. I think there are two reasons for this.

Firstly, although this was an incredibly important speaking situation for me was never nervous about it. I've been incredibly busy this last week and I have never even thought twice about the speech this morning. This is something I would have been dreading for months in advance before the Programme, but now I barely thought twice about it. I think this is an incredible thing because it shows i have removed most of the stress I used to associate with speaking. I have the confidence to know I can handle any speaking situation and this is enough for me to just do it. So doing it wasn't as a big a deal as I thought it would be.

Secondly, although my technique was good and I feel my eloquence was high in most of the speech there were still a couple of wobbles at the end. These were really just a lack of preparation (again, because I had been busy and not been dreading the speech I hadn't spent ages preparing) and any slight wobble I had I went back to cancel immediately (that only happened once). Out of 5mins, 4 minutes and 55 seconds was very good and eloquent, but 5 second at the end was a bit bumpy (but still not stuttering). Rather than focus on the 4 minutes, 55 seconds of great speech as well as the occasion itself and the self-disclosure in the content of the speech I instead chose to focus on the 5 seconds of slight bumpiness at the end. I didn't allow myself to enjoy the moment afterwards. I feel I am a bit of a perfectionist now with my speech.

This in itself says a lot. I never thought as a stutter that I would ever become a perfectionist with my speech! Rather than falling into the fluency trap I feel I sometimes fall into the trap of being a proud instructor. I feel that because I am an instructor I should always speak 100% as strong as I do in McGuire courses. I feel that unless my technique is 100% all the time then I've failed. Any small mistake I make I beat myself up about it. After speaking to two people after the event they said that being a good example is not about being, 100% eloquent in every situation (this was my hardest situation yet) but rather in being honest, canceling, not avoiding, using support etc. I know all this already, but it's sometimes hard to see it yourself. Blinkers, etc.

I was probably too hard on myself because this was an incredible situation for me. Listening back to my Dictaphone I'm trying to step back and see the bigger picture about what i have achieved. That is why I am now on Cloud Number 9. The speech did go very well and I feel fantastic that I have been able to do this after so long. Thank you for the people who helped me see that and also who helped me warm up. George Samios, Alan Wyatt, Terry Cardwell, Stephen Harte, Gareth Gates, Stephen Fletcher and everyone who has been supportive of me doing this in the past couple of weeks. Its this support, which made me motivate myself to do this speech and then also realize what a great thing I had done once I did it. Thank you.

I'm off round the world for a year as of this Saturday, so this is a great thing to really remove some of my old baggage before I go traveling. It's a nightmare having excess baggage in a foreign country, particularly getting on trains.

Cheers for listening!

Story from South Australia

by Robert Lucas (Australia)

My name is Robert Lucas. I was on the McGuire Programme on January 1999. I was a bad stutterer, who would shy away from every speaking situation, using every trick I could. My whole life was one of avoidances and only making friends through my wife and other friends.

When I first arrived in Sydney I was very nervous and apprehensive about what was going to happen to me on this course. I had tried everything from Hypnotherapy to smooth speech, although they seemed to help at the time, they had no long term effect and the let down was they did not have any support afterwards.

When we assembled that Wednesday to do our first day Videos my heart was racing like a run away train. My turn came and I was adamant that I was going to get my proper name out, not the name I called myself (Bob). I came away from the videoing thinking to myself that I had done a great job in hiding my stutter. When I saw it sometime afterwards, I did not realize how severe my stutter was. I still watch it now and then, to enforce within myself that I never want to be like that again.

Simon Bailey was the course Instructor. To me the first day was very intense, where you where shown the new breathing technique and how to wear your belt, this, with the checklist was repeated over and over. We were to learn afterwards that this was the most important part of the course. That night we were encouraged to stand up and say our name and address, a situation I would try to avoid at all costs. I held back from going first and watched in disbelief as other students around stood up and said their name with confidence and without stuttering. Now I couldn't wait to stand up myself and when my time came everything I said was with perfect technique and without that silly stutter, my ears where listening to the words that I had wanted to say for fifty years – *my name.*

What really opened up my eyes to this wonderful way of speaking was going out with a coach to do contacts. My coach showed me all the ways to make contacts. Walking down one of the Sydney streets with him it suddenly dawned on me this is what it was all about. Facing your fears to talk and approach as many people as you could, from that time onwards all the speaking fear faded away.

The next day we got the introduction to the Harrison workshop that showed us, you could have fun with your speech and then it was our turn to do contacts with the coaches. I was pacing myself with the number of contacts I made. This was easy with the help of my coach. I was talking to people that I would never dream of speaking to. Then came the public speech at Circular Quay, this was the biggest fear I had to face, not that I was frightened of stuttering as I could now control it, but it was the fear of facing a large crowd of people, who were looking at me. Up I got, out came the words, no stuttering, everyone was looking, I made as much eye contact with different people as I could, everything went OK. I got down and felt like a new person. One that was not afraid to speak anywhere, anytime and without stuttering. Wow! What a feeling.

The rest of the course went by and it was time to go home to Adelaide. My wife picked me up at the airport, and to impress her I took her over to the car rental counter and did a disclosure, looking back at her I saw the joy and tears in her eyes. We both knew that I was on the road to really conquering my stutter and start enjoying speaking … and my life.

It's been a long road and is still a long road, with lots of little detours that you have to be careful of, because these can lead you to the swamp. Since doing the Course, I have learnt more about myself and how people perceived me, than during my whole life.

I have faced all my fears, joined speaking clubs, stand up comedy, made speeches at work, done TV interviews, radio interviews, and joined a drama class to gain even more confidence. These days I look forward to facing any challenge handed to me.

Although I still stumble at times I know where I have gone wrong and these days it does not worry me as it used to. I maintain that you must have commitment and without this you will take that detour to the swamp. One of my biggest thrills was to be selected by Dave McGuire to be a Regional Evaluator.

Another great satisfaction was to be chosen as Team Leader on the Adelaide 4 day intensive.

I am in the McGuire Programme to help myself, whilst helping other stutterers.

The Welsh teacher

By Kevin Phelps (Wales)

My name is Kevin Phelps. I live in Wales, UK.

I joined the McGuire Programme in August 1999 attending my first course in Harrogate, North Yorkshire.

For 7 years before joining the Programme I had been working as a Primary School Teacher. I coped because for me speaking in front of children, where they don't judge your skills of communication, doesn't carry much fear. Somehow I got by. Although meetings, phone calls and more formal situations e.g. training courses, parent evenings etc. involving adult interaction was at times extremely difficult.

After 5 years I applied for a job as a Deputy Head of a school. Primarily because the job was in Pembrokeshire, Britain's only Coastal National Park, in South West Wales. It is the area I originally came from. A beautiful place that I had to leave to find a job initially but now wanted to move back to raise my family.

I was short listed for interview but stuttered so much in the interview that I asked on two occasions if I could leave, eventually I walked out. I was extremely upset and distressed not only because I had seriously embarrassed and humiliated myself but also I knew I'd never be able to pass any future interviews and therefore never be able to move back to Pembrokeshire. It was that experience that prompted me to research 'Stuttering and My Stutter' and I eventually discovered the McGuire Programme.

After a few courses and loads of hard work and significant improvement over the control in my speech I felt ready for another interview for a Deputy Headship. One came up in May 2000 and I decided to go for it. The interview involved me giving a presentation for 10 minutes and then being interviewed extremely formally by a panel of 15 people, the full governing body of the school. A nightmare scenario for even any non-stutterer.

However, it was different this time. I was totally educated by the McGuire Programme. I had disclosed in my application form that I was a someone trying to overcome a stutter, I prepared for the interview by warming up with strong Costal breathing (the technique I had learned on the McGuire courses), I telephoned my coaches before the interview and put myself into a very positive mindset. During the interview I used good eye contact, I smiled and paused and all in all gave a strong, confident and thoughtful interview. I just knew it had gone well.

The result was that I was informed soon after, thanks to the McGuire Programme, that the 15 interviewers had voted unanimously for me and the job was mine.

Finally, I was able to move to Pembrokeshire with my wife and children (two boys, Toby and Joe) and build our dream home very close to the Pembrokeshire Coast. Stuttering was not going to hold me back anymore.

Since then, I have maintained my contact with the McGuire

Programme and have graduated through the Programme to become a Telephone Coach, a Course Instructor (I am instructing my third course this year) and a Staff Trainer. This has allowed me great opportunities to further develop my own speaking skills as well as the wonderful work of helping other people out of the misery of out of control stuttering.

It is now 2007, nine years since my first course. In this time I have done numerous radio and newspaper interviews, a TV interview, countless lectures, presentations, performed as an after dinner speaker you name it!!!

Just over a year ago I was successful in gaining my first Headship in the teaching profession. Life goes on ...

Thanks to the McGuire Programme I really have been given a new life!!!

My experience

By Bill Fabian (Australia)

It's been nearly four years now since I attended my first McGuire Programme course in Sydney in February 1999. I am now able to reflect back on the person I was before that time and who I am now.

In the past I had a couple of situations in which I felt comfortable with my speech. This was particularly true of speech pathology clinics. Outside these few situations I would often experience spasms in my speech that were so severe that I would feel debilitated and totally non-functional. I still have occasional blocks but they are just glitches which are dealt with and then I move on. The uncertainty of falling into a chasm from which there was no escape has gone.

All the joys of life in the past had a shadow cast over them. I found it difficult to really enjoy life, despite the fact that I tried very hard to be happy by intent and accept myself as a person who stutters. It was like an ever-present black cloud hanging over me that just wouldn't go away. My hidden underlying view of life was 'One day I'll be dead and I won't have to suffer this torment anymore.' I now feel very content with myself and just have to deal with all those other frustrations that are common to everyone. Life is good.

I was a very heavy drinker in the past. Just about every night I'd polish off a bottle of some alcoholic beverage. Luckily I was not a physically addicted alcoholic but just used it to numb the pain. It was what I used to chill-out and find some peace and contentment for a while. It also seemed to help my speech but I now realize this was an illusion. Now I don't touch a drop. Alcohol causes me to get out of touch with myself and I really find value in being fully self-aware. The savings in not buying alcohol has compensated for the cost of the course many times over.

In the past my wife always made the inquiries when a telephone call had to be made or when making a joint purchase. It's not that I couldn't do it. It was just that there didn't seem to be much point in my going through the struggle when there was an easy way out. I now do most of the talking when we are in joint speaking situations.

I often used 'ah' and 'um' as a crutch in the past. When I was asked for my name it would most times be 'Umb-umb-umb-umBill Arf-arf-arf-arf-arFabian.' I have now eliminated that trick and speak in a much more eloquent style. I had quite a few physical 'helpers' in the past to get my words out. Everything from a leg slap to a knee dip. These tricks looked very undignified and were behaviors that were really out of my control in the heat of the moment. Needless to say, they are all now gone.

In the past I would find myself in situations where it was easier to remain silent in the background rather than draw attention to myself. There really is no place to hide though and there would always be some-one who would say, 'You're very quiet.' My reply would be, 'I've got nothing to say.' This was a lie of course and I now have no problems in making my thoughts known.

I would often break out in sweat and go cherry red in the face when I was caught up in a strenuous blocking episode. Sometimes this would even result in my glasses fogging up in certain climatic conditions. These days I'm calm, cool and collected in most situations. I certainly don't 'sweat it' any more.

At times in the past I had a very small voice. Unconsciously, sometimes I would whisper or just mouth the words I wanted to say. Now I can produce a strong and powerful voice when I need to with very little effort.

Fear and dread would often accompany me when I approached speaking situations. The anticipation was sometimes worse than the act of speaking itself. I now approach speaking situations with enthusiasm and still get a kick out of being able to walk into a shop and ask for what I want in the knowledge that I can do so with clarity.

In the past I would sometimes experienced periods of effortless fluency; the so-called 'fluency ride'. I really enjoyed these times but inevitably they never lasted very long and when I came down, I came down hard. I now have consistency in my speech and the uncertainty of not knowing what to expect next has gone.

I tried all the traditional therapies that were available and even though they seemed to alleviate my problems for a while they never provided a long term solution. They worked very well in the speech clinic but I could never successfully integrate the methods into my speaking personality. In some ways they even added to the feeling of holding back. Now if I just manage my thoughts, feelings and emotions the rest of the things I do to retain confident, forward moving speech just fall into place. The thought that I use to quickly muster my resources is 'Stand tall, think tall, talk tall.'

Despite trying to accept myself as a person who stutters in the past, I still felt a degree of shame in my condition. I now have pride in myself irrespective of the condition of my speech. The first time I attended Toastmasters and was asked to introduce myself I did so by replicating my very worst blocking behavior, with all the secondaries. I then paused, looked into the eyes of my audience and with eloquence and confidence, explained what stuttering is and how I was dealing with it. In my time in Toastmasters, three people independently approached me to ask if I could teach them to put more power into their delivery.

All in all, life was pretty tough for me before 1999. The only regret that I have with the McGuire Programme was that it wasn't available five years earlier. This was a pivotal period in my life and when the going got tough I could not get going. This period culminated in a time of career change and opportunity, which will never come again. I blew it and almost ended up having a nervous breakdown in the process. How different things would have been if I had gained the skills I have now have a few years earlier.

Despite all the success I have experienced in recent years I still consider myself to be a person who stutters or at least one with the potential to stutter. I don't know if that mindset will ever leave me, as I still have 40 years of identity to deal with. Perhaps I really don't want to just be a fluent speaker and perhaps being a person who has prevailed over the debilitating condition that stuttering can be, is more than enough. I know for sure that the old speaking personality that handicapped me so much in the past is now dead and buried.

I'm always happy to speak to anyone about the McGuire Programme and in fact about anything at all. Please feel free to contact me at willf999@yahoo.com and I'll send you my phone number.

My journey

by Joe O Donnell (Ireland)
At the age of three, I developed a stutter. And like most kids who developed a stutter at that age, it didn't become a major problem for me until several years later. When I started to build up my vocabulary, I found out that I could substitute easy to say words for difficult words. It was about that time that I felt and knew that I was totally different from the other boys of my age simply because I became very hesitant in delivering my speech and would often say phrases that had no meaning. Apart from that I looked no different than Mickey next door. This led me to become very confused whether I was in a group or by myself. After every verbal encounter I would walk away, my eyes fixated on the ground, praying that it would open up and devour me so that I would never have to face another verbal encounter again and feel in my chest the confusion on my listeners face. I would end up trying to replay in my mind what I had actually said and more often than not I ended up really hating myself for saying the oddest things, lying and being the coward that I was.

Being a covert stutterer, I never had to roll a word about in my mouth for ten seconds. I didn't have all that facial and body struggle that most people associate with stutterers. All I did was avoid words. No big deal? At that time people didn't know that I stuttered, simply because I never stuttered in front of them. I would scan ahead for any negative emotional words, open up my in-built dictionary, picked the easiest one to say that would relate to the word that I avoided.

I was disgusted with myself at what I had done but I kept my most sacred secret intact. I knew that they sensed that something was not right with me. They couldn't quite understand the reasoning in my fluent responses and that lead them to believe that I was either very stupid or had lost the plot completely.

I knew that neither was the case. If only I could make myself struggle like those so very lucky overt stutterers, and then I could prove them wrong. But my lack of courage was much more powerful than my determination to be one of the lucky ones, so I opted for a life of avoidances in order to hang on to my secret.

Out of the frying pan and into the fire.
The opportunity arose when I was sixteen years old to be the third generation of O'Donnells to join the highly respected family butcher business. My prayers were answered.

Free at last from the clutches of my sneering peer group. I would never have to sit in classroom and soak up time after time my hidden tears of humiliation. There was a god after all. Then I realized that I had just spent my last ten years or so living my suspended life sentence in an open prison and now the time had come to pay my price to society. Solitary confinement. What seemed like a blunt knife tearing my chest to pieces was now only a thorn in my finger compared to what I was to encounter.

I had to get away from '*how much*', '*what does that weigh*', and most of all '*can you answer the telephone*'. Those three phrases remained with me for years. I wasn't very good at being a butcher. A butcher needs to be friendly, needs to be able to communicate in order to sell his produce, needs to know the hind quarter from the four quarter and needs to be able to sharpen his knife and keep it sharp. I could do none of the above. Once again I felt that I had failed in life. I would have been quite happy, if circumstances had been different, to get a job that didn't require talking.

But loyalty was such a huge part of me and cowardice was even stronger so I persevered 24/7.

Path to Freedom
I finally made the move to make my escape from solitary confinement to enjoying the sound of approaching voices and ringing

telephones thanks to Patrick Merrigan, Maree Sweeney and Victoria Bradshaw. They showed me the path to freedom. They shared with me how they, through hard work, perseverance and initially a little bearable pain, had got rid of their plunging knife and replaced it with the odd thorn in their finger. I hope to reach my destination too, but I need to keep on this road and live by the same rules as all those who have already reached theirs. Thanks to David McGuire for sharing his Programme with us, for all those brave people who helped me and countless others on this journey and for my better half Alice who supported and still supports me 100% of her time. Even if I never reach my destination, the most important thing is that I am enjoying the journey.

The briefing

By Lance Austin (Australia)

Where I work, Monday Afternoon Briefing is a regular event, and the chance to present a *lot* of information in a very *little* bit of time; hence, time pressure and pace are often necessary evils. Yesterday, Monday (09 September 2002), I 'pushed that ol' envelope' and delivered my first *(fluent!)* briefing at work, for many, many years.

Our 'loving/kind' Director, apparently impressed with my performance two weeks earlier (see below), was determined he wanted to see a *real* presentation from me on one of my *real* work issues; well, I wrote it, gave it, it was good, and I was fluent and in control (!). I even stuck in a big use Deliberate Dysfluency in the middle, and it worked. The TWO MINUTE briefing (I'm not joking! That's all the time you get!) was the first hurdle, then came the Director's question: That was the hard part! Pause, analyze, clarify, formulate, and don't verbal 'tap dance' too much with the answer, the most important thing.

Being first up was also a bit of a nail-biter, but it allowed me to stand there, take my time, start when I wanted to, and be seen as a credible speaker, as well as a credible analyst ...ironically, yesterday was even harder, than the briefing I gave two weeks earlier to a packed house of two hundred (!!!!!!) I had decided to brief on the McGuire Programme Course conducted in July here in Sydney, the outcomes, and what it meant for me, so it amounted to a full-on disclosure to the whole organization.

I had the blessing of my bosses, and the stage was set. I was last out of six people briefing, so I was so afraid that my heart was pounding like ...a great, big pounding thing! Yet, once I began, I gave the most powerful, in control, and fluent presentation I have ever, ever given. At the end, I also made my recommendations that all of the Defence Organisation and all uniformed military members with a stuttering problem should be given ample access to the McGuire Programme.

Even weeks before, I would have not *dared* to step up on that stage (!), to speak to so many powerful people – Colonels, One Star Generals, and other senior Defence civilians of Two-Star rank. The liberated feeling was overwhelming, and the emails of praise that afternoon kept coming. I even cried at home with my wife that evening; I was stunned at how positive the whole experience was ...and wished that the feeling could have lasted forever.

Keep your faith, Freedom's Road-Sters, work hard, and keep your faith! My successes I've relayed to you here, still don't stop me blocking with that pretty girl at the bakery, or the nice bloke/guy at my local pizzeria. But remember: When you get a block that seizes up the whole chest, and you feel you can't say the first word you want to, and choose another word, *go back* to that same person later – not someone else, the *same person* – and do a proper disclosure/cancellation. Ask for that thing, you couldn't say before, and ask for it as many times as you feel you need to. That person, if a *good* person, will think you are so cool, and so brave! It's good for you, it restores your self-respect, and you aren't cheating yourself in the long term at least.

Battling

by Patrick Merrigan (Ireland)

It is eighteen weeks since my first course in Glasgow, Sept. 1996. I've had a battle with a feared word 'Sutton' for some time now. I believed I had it licked. I was wrong. Six weeks after Glasgow I took a big fall ... a crash. I had been invited to say a few words at a social business gathering in October and looked forward to it with a little trepidation. Some time before the evening dinner and after the pageantry, I was told by the golf club President that I wouldn't be speaking. Disappointment but joy, I could relax for the evening ... my mistake. I turned off my motor (Costal breathing) and reverted spontaneously to my former comfortable discomfort ... tricks, avoidance etc. During the dinner and after not a few glasses of dry white, the President approached me: 'Paddy, we're starting the speeches soon, you will say a few words?' Oh my God I'm thinking, what's happening? My heart pounding thinking 'I can't do it; I'll make a fool of myself before the press and my client'. All the old fears came up, confusion and panic. I plucked the courage to go to the president and to my terrible shame, guilt and feeling a total jackass, I lied through my teeth –'I have to go home urgently, due to a family matter'. I got my assistant to do the excuses for me and disappeared through the side door like a thief in the night. Hating myself for deserting the battle and beating my head above the left ear with my fist, I drove for four hours.

What am I? Where am I going in my life? 'I can't handle this Programme' I thought. I really would prefer being dead. I was back on my old suicide road again. I telephoned Dave the following morning, Monday, and after a short period, had me breathing and advised I must cancel what I had done and get back in training.

On Wednesday of that week, I walked into Toastmasters alone. With a feeling that must be similar to going to the guillotine, I requested the person taking the money at the entrance, that I would like the opportunity to speak— this being my first time speaking and that I was a someone trying to overcome a stutter. I won the table topics award that evening. Had lost a major battle at Tullamore, but countered with a win at Toastmasters. I have won a second award since.

The battle with Sutton was not over though. Wednesday three days ago, at a formal business meeting, I was again anxious about the feared 'Sutton'. During the meeting it came up in my mouth again. I was playing 'not to lose', instead of 'playing to win'. I was flagellating, feeling I shouldn't be here. My hexagon again plummeted, the enemy the stuttering monster was back. I kept my outward composure while inside I was dying. Must get back on the street immediately and to hell with meetings and dinner. It was 9:15 p.m. in Cork.

At about 11 p.m. and having lost count with the number of situations some of them repeated to the same people with the question: 'excuse me (pause), can you tell me, (pause), where is (pause), ssss ... su ... sut Sutton House?' It wasn't getting much better, but no avoidance. I decided I might probably be up all night but the streets were getting quiet and I had met the same policeman twice. I was quite desperate but scrapping and fighting. I was not going home to a sleepless night. I tried to telephone Conor but he was engaged. Went through my checklist. Try one more item. Deep through the chest, it worked instantly, 'the greater the fear the deeper the voice'. I had five or six perfect hits. My hexagon was coming up good. Entered a full pub and with a powerful 'excuse me please' the whole pub turned to the door. Just about everybody in the pub knew where Sutton House was. Same with the pub next door. One hour earlier, I had great difficulty stuttering out 'Sutton' to a drunk on the street. Celebrated with a Chinese and couple of glasses of dry white. I liked and respected myself and had done my best and I suspect the dour look had left my face. I felt great. Telephoned Robert to tell him he had saved me with 'deep through the chest' but I knew the enemy would be waiting for me the following morning. Called Dave at 6 a.m., thankfully he wasn't in his bath and I dismissed the guilty feeling of his skin becoming prune like during our extended telephone exchange. (One of the things about this Programme are the gigantic telephone bills. Believe me, they are your lifeline and mandatory)

I had choices to make and had arranged meetings away on Friday, Saturday and Sunday. Wasn't much point going to business meetings in my negative hexagon condition. I decided to cancel and re-schedule my plans. Back on the street Thursday at 10.30 am in Cork still looking for that elusive and lost Sutton House. Wasn't coming out good, though I was deep through the chest. Damn it, what next. I persevered with 60 situations and headed for a meeting nearby at 2.30 p.m. with people over from the UK whom I hadn't met before. I had a 45-minute drive and again was searching the CHECKLIST. Fast and Full, Hmmmmm. Let's try a few to myself in the car and on the recorder. Doesn't sound good. Faster and fuller (Costal breath). I think I'm pausing at the bottom where the Diaphragm has gone from all the way up to all the way down with poor timing and a poor first sound. I stopped the car and drilled for ten minutes. I think I have it, let's find a scalp to take.

Stopped a man in his car, waved him down (little narrow country road) so I could see the reflection in his eye. Expelled residual air, eye contact, good perceptions, fired my now well rehearsed question. Bulls eye. Perfect. Thank you. Let's find a few more scalps and test the remodeled speech. Perfect hit after hit. Went to my meeting and use Deliberate Dysfluency with the best Caselton 'smooth and slow' I could muster. I found my speech speeding up, must slow down. I was back again and liked myself even better.

Day three, Friday, time to overkill. Hit the street at 10.30 am, did another 70 and a little shopping and had fun. It's now 3.15 pm and I can honestly say I did my best and boy was it worth the pain. It's great. I forgot to mention that I had already done 200 or so situations on *Sutton* before the Dublin course and thought I had it licked. Wrong. Dave says it takes thirty days to break a habit. I think maybe it takes 500–600 or more situations to really kill your most feared word. But this is assuming you aren't reinforcing the old habit at the same time.

Bad News

There will be times when you may be scared to death and have choices to make. To become a fearless warrior, you must have skirmishes and fight many battles. Each battle makes you a better warrior, though painful it may be. Do not run away, it is much more difficult to return to the battlefield, if at all you return. You have choices, to go back to prison for life or fight the monster and set you free. Only you can do it. The sooner you practice Deliberate Dysfluency. and expose yourself as a someone trying to overcome a stutter the shorter the Road to Freedom.

Good News

Battle scarred and victorious, you can hold your head high with the best of them, though you are probably better in speaking terms. You will keep your head, trust yourself develop patience and a greater understanding of yourself and others. You will understand the real meaning of honesty and integrity and yet have an air of the Old Western Cowboys who says little but when they do, everybody listens. Above all you will have dignity, self respect and be able to handle just about anything that comes your way.

The home of the soul

By Rakan Otaibi (Middle East)

'The ancient Greeks called the diaphragm 'the home of the soul' and since I learned breathing from the diaphragm to control my stutter, I started to speak from my soul rather than from my false ego.'
SALAM ALIKOM

For as long as I can remember I've stuttered and throughout my life I have tried numerous techniques to overcome it, even I developed stuttering fast with secondary behaviors like substituting words, tightening body muscles. Speaking was the toughest job for me.

When the course instructor in the first day video asked me about my family I said eight members because it was difficult to say four I could not say I have four young lovely sisters. It's really painful for a young intelligent man to stream his ideas, thoughts, opinions and emotions only into paper and texts.

After attending my first course I realized It's not about becoming fluent, it's about acceptance and making the most out of life, no chains, no mountain crushing me, smiling, laughing, coaching graduates, listening to people, pat somebody's back and give someone high five. To me that's what I called being cured.

Reading list

Denis Waitley, *The New Dynamics of Winning* (Gain the mind-set of a champion). London, Nicholas Brealey Publishing, 1994.
Denis talks about all those qualities it takes to accomplish your goals and win the tournament of life. He makes many references to successfull athletes and business people.

Peter McWilliams, *Do it! Let's Get Off Our Buts . . .* London, HarperCollins, 2001.
Like the title says, it's time to stop making excuses for failure – stop the 'buts.' He, too, talks about the importance of just getting down to work.

Tim Gallwey, *The Inner Game of Tennis*. London, Pan Macmillan, 1986.
This book will give you greater insight into the whys of focal point and imaging the diaphragm. It is one of the best books on getting out of your own way and letting your body (including your speaking mechanism) do what it knows how to do.

Manuel Smith, *When I Say No, I Feel Guilty*. New York, Bantam, 1975.
The original textbook on assertiveness training. Assertiveness is the opposite of holding back and avoidance. Holding back in one part of your life can easily lead to holding back in speaking. Holding back and avoiding is the psychological core of stammering.

Rogers and McMillin, *Relapse Traps*. New York, Bantam, 1992.
Because of the addictive qualities of tricks and avoidance, a stutterer will relapse for the same reason a substance abuser will relapse. It is important for you to recognize these traps.

Susan Jeffers, *Feel The Fear and Do It Anyway*. London, Random House, 1992.
Great book on dealing with those 'negative tapes' and getting out of your comfort zone. You have to get out of your comfort zone to win the war against stammering.

John Harrison, *How to Conquer Your Fears of Speaking Before People*, Order it directly from: John Harrison, e: John@thewriterstouch.com Phone (415) 647 4700.
I met John in 1995 at the World Congress on stammering in Sweden. He opened new doors for me personally as well as for my Programme. He won the war against his own stammer by taking care of those other places in his life where he was holding back. He did this through hard work ... doing what he learned from growth workshops and books

Books by members of the Programme.

Sue Cottrell *'Can I tell you about Stammering?'* for Jessica Kingsley Publishers, 2013.

Michael O'Shea *'Why I Called My Sister Harry'* Trafford

Index